the prostate

small gland **big** problem

third edition

by Roger S Kirby MA MD FRCS (Urol) FEBU

Professor of Urology

Director, The Prostate Centre, London

Chairman, Prostate Research Campaign UK

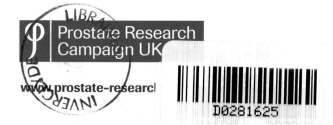

The prostate: small gland, big problem
First published 2000
Second edition 2002
Third edition 2006

© 2006 Prostate Research Campaign UK

Prostate Research Campaign UK (Registered Charity No. 1037063) aims to provide information, promote education and raise funds to finance scientific and medical research into prostate disorders. Donations to further these aims may be sent to Prostate Research Campaign UK, 10 Northfields Prospect, Putney Bridge Road, London SW18 1PE, UK. Tel: 020 8877 2609

Published by Prostate Research Campaign UK (www.prostate-research.org.uk) in association with Health Press Limited, Elizabeth House, Queen Street, Abingdon, Oxon OX14 3LN, UK. Tel: 01235 523233

A note on gender
Please note that we refer to doctors throughout this book as 'he'. This in no way reflects any bias against female practitioners – this step has been taken merely to avoid clumsiness. We trust that female GPs and urologists will realize that no offence is intended and take none.

A CIP record for this title is available from the British Library.

ISBN 1-903734-89-4 (978-903734-89-6)

Kirby, RS (Roger)
The prostate: small gland, big problem/
Roger S Kirby

Illustrated by Dee McLean, MeDee Art, London, UK.

Cover design by Kevin Hinton
Typeset by Zed, Oxford
Printed by LinneyPrint Ltd, Mansfield, UK.

Dedicated to the memory of
SHEILA KILMISTER
1935–2006
"Love is, above all, the gift of oneself"

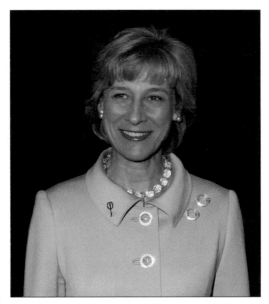

**Her Royal Highness
The Duchess of Gloucester, GCVO**

From HRH The Duchess of Gloucester, GCVO

It is good news that the third edition of Professor Roger Kirby's excellent book on prostate-related problems and treatment is now ready – revised and updated to the last minute on knowledge and guidance. The second edition is only a few years old, but medical science, not least within urology, moves so fast and the treatments for both prostate cancer and other prostate-related disorders have greatly advanced over the last four years.

Although I understand that it is much valued by the medical profession, this textbook is aimed at us, the lay readers, and I congratulate Professor Kirby on his ability to write comprehensively and in such a straightforward way on a highly complex subject. Having consulted these pages, any patient with a prostate problem, or anyone concerned for him, should be left in no doubt that the immediate next step must be to consult a doctor.

In my few years as Patron of Prostate Research Campaign UK, I have learnt that time is of the essence, and I cannot emphasise enough that the sooner a problem, or even a suspicion of something not quite right, is dealt with, the greater the chance of recovery. The statistics are really encouraging for a return to a full bill of health when a prostate problem is not allowed to develop but is confronted and corrected without delay.

Acknowledgements

Prostate Research Campaign UK would like to thank
Mandy Klyne and Health Press for editorial assistance,
Kevin Hinton at the Blake Project for designing the cover,
Dee McLean for the illustrations, and Jane Dawoodi and
Clive Turner for their contributions to earlier editions
on which this book is based. Thanks are also due to
LinneyPrint Ltd for their financial contribution to printing.

www.prostate-research.org.uk

Contents

Introduction

At the beginning of the 20th century, the average life expectancy for a man in Europe or the USA was a mere 49 years. As diseases of the prostate typically affect men beyond middle age, the likelihood of a man in the early 1900s suffering from one of these conditions was rather slim. Now, at the dawn of the new millennium, however, life expectancy for men extends well into the 70s, and this increased longevity has been accompanied by a rising tide of prostate disease. Over the next 20 years, life expectancy is predicted to rise still further, to 80 and beyond. What we are witnessing at the moment is, then, simply the tip of the iceberg. The number of men with a prostate problem is set to more than double by the year 2020.

Recently there has been a surge in public interest in the prostate, largely as the result of a spate of media attention. Scarcely a week goes by without a newspaper or television feature on this aspect of men's health. Prominent personalities, including the former Archbishop of Canterbury Lord Runcie, Sir Harry Secombe and George Carman QC, have also spoken openly about their prostate problems before, sadly, passing away as a result of the disease.

This increasing focus can only be good news, as men with prostate disease can increase their chance of cure with a little knowledge and timely action. Men, and their partners and family who love and support them, need to be aware of the symptoms and signs of prostate problems, and the possibilities of a simple examination and a blood and/or urine test. The third edition of this book contains the essence of the things that you and those closest to you need to know to respond appropriately to the threat of these widespread diseases. Use this information to obtain the best treatment for you – you owe it to yourself and to those who are dear to you.

How you can help yourself

Men's attitude towards their health has traditionally been 'if it ain't broke, don't fix it'. These days, the thinking should be more along the lines of 'if you look after your body (and particularly your heart and your prostate), it has less of a tendency to go wrong'.

Seeing your doctor

All three prostate diseases – prostate cancer, benign prostatic hyperplasia (BPH) and prostatitis – tend to have a greater impact on a sufferer's quality of life than is, in fact, necessary. These conditions frequently reach a relatively advanced stage before men seek medical help, which is often the result of men's *laissez-faire* attitude to lower urinary tract symptoms, embarrassment about discussing this area of their anatomy with their doctor, and their general reluctance to undergo and act on regular health checks.

In fact, each of the three major prostatic diseases eloquently illustrates the 'stitch in time' principle. A 'window of curability' exists for prostate cancer, but once this is closed, neither surgery nor radiotherapy is likely, ultimately, to be successful. With BPH, several studies have confirmed that there is a level of secondary damage to the bladder caused by obstruction after which complete recovery becomes less likely. And if prostatitis becomes chronic, then repeated and prolonged courses of treatment are often needed.

Regarding prostate health, regular prostate checks allow disease to be detected at a stage when it can generally be resolved, while preventive strategies may reduce the risks of disease developing in the first place. It makes good sense to combine these with regular, more general health checks to diagnose other potentially dangerous conditions such as high blood pressure, lipid disorders and diabetes. In a sense then, the prostate provides the key to more general men's health.

Points to remember

- If men wait for symptoms, they wait too long

- Men with prostate disease can be cured by a little knowledge and timely action

- A 'window of curability' exists for prostate cancer

- If cancer is to be identified at a stage when it is still curable, then it should be detected before the PSA rises much above 10 ng/mL

- More than 80% of men who have had a radical prostatectomy are alive 10 years afterwards, and 60% are alive at 15 years

- With a radical prostatectomy, the success rate in removing the tumour and preventing recurrence is commonly over 80%

- If cancer is present, it can stay dormant, grow slowly or accelerate rapidly, for reasons that are not yet fully understood

Lifestyle

Adopting a healthier lifestyle, in terms of both diet and exercise, is obviously desirable. By staying slim and fit, you are more likely to remain healthy and, in particular, you will reduce your chances of developing cardiovascular disease and diabetes. This may also benefit your prostate, as there is increasing evidence that overweight men and men with higher cholesterol levels are more susceptible to prostate cancer. BPH is also more common in obese men and surgery in obese individuals is more risky. Finally, prostatitis will often resolve as general health improves. In prostate disease, as in so many other areas, prevention is better than cure.

Diet

A healthy diet is essential for good health, and the best way to achieve this is to eat moderate quantities of a wide variety of the right foods. Try to eat or drink:

- less fat, particularly saturated fats, which are found in fatty meats and dairy products, and 'trans fats', which are found mostly in margarine and processed baked goods
- more fish and chicken (but not the skin), and less red meat
- plenty of fresh fruit and vegetables – try and eat *at least* five portions and aim for nine portions a day (see page 110)
- foods high in fibre, such as wholewheat bread and grains
- less sugar and salt
- moderate amounts of tea, coffee and alcohol.

Exercise

Regular exercise is essential for good health and plays an important role in reducing the risk of developing many diseases. A recent study in America found that men who undertook 3 hours of vigorous exercise per week were 70% less likely to develop or die from prostate cancer. Exercise also helps us to maintain a healthy body weight, particularly when combined with a healthy diet. The prominent 'beer belly' that is so characteristic of overweight men is strongly linked to an increased risk of heart attack and stroke. It therefore makes sense to try to do some moderate physical exercise for at least 30 minutes five times or more a week. Remember that vigorous exercise not only burns off calories as you do it, but also increases the metabolic rate for several hours after the exertion.

Smoking

Those readers who smoke are strongly exhorted to give it up! Although smoking does not cause prostate disease directly, it may result in bladder and kidney cancer and, because it damages blood vessels, it may also result in reduced erections and sexual dysfunction.

Maintaining prostate health

Minerals

Selenium has been shown to reduce the incidence of all cancers and prostate cancer in particular. It is found in grains, nuts and oily fish but, because the soil in the UK contains low

5

levels of selenium, the average intake in this country is well below the recommended amount. You can increase your intake either by eating three or four Brazil nuts every day or by taking one of the many supplements that are widely available in a dose of 200 micrograms a day.

Zinc deficiency is unusual, but may be responsible for some prostate problems, as well as impotence. It is therefore important to include good sources of zinc in your diet, like meat, fish, whole grains and legumes, such as peas and beans.

Antioxidants

Antioxidants are thought to protect the body's cells against cancer-causing substances. The main antioxidants, which are found in fruit and vegetables, are vitamins A, C and E, and lycopene, which is found in tomatoes. The two most effective antioxidants are vitamin E and lycopene.

Vitamin E. Taking a vitamin E supplement has been shown to reduce deaths from prostate cancer by about 40%. However, trials investigating vitamin E supplements showed an increase in deaths, possibly as a result of cardiovascular problems, in those taking a dose of more than 150 International Units (IU) per day. It has therefore been suggested that the daily dose of vitamin E be restricted to 150 International Units (IU) per day, which has not been associated with such problems.

Tomatoes contain abundant quantities of lycopene, which is one of the most powerful antioxidants. Research has shown that those people who eat a lot of tomatoes and tomato products have a lower risk of certain cancers, particularly prostate cancer. Tomatoes are more effective when they have been processed or cooked, because heating with a little oil helps to release the lycopene from the tomato skin and makes it easier to absorb.

Cranberry juice

Urinary tract infections are more common in men with an enlarged prostate gland. While such infections are not life-threatening or significant, they can have a considerable financial and social toll on those affected. Although more research is needed, drinking one or two glasses of cranberry juice a day does seem to ward off urinary tract infections in some individuals. A word of caution: if you are taking warfarin, you should avoid cranberry juice as it can potentiate the effects of the drug.

Blueberry juice is thought to have similar properties and is also an antioxidant. Highly coloured fruits such as strawberries are also recommended.

Saw palmetto

The herb saw palmetto (*Serenoa repens*) is a plant native to the south-east of the USA. It has been shown to inhibit the action of 5-alpha-reductase (see page 80), growth factors and inflammatory substances responsible for the common symptoms of BPH (see page 75). A recent study reported in the *New England Journal of Medicine* called into doubt its efficacy; however, some patients swear by it, so more research is needed.

Other therapies

A host of other complementary therapies are claimed to protect against prostate cancer, but sound evidence for their safety and efficacy is sparse. This includes soya products, green tea, apricot kernels, pomegranates and St John's wort. Cancer patients, in particular, are very vulnerable to hype about so-called 'alternative' therapies, many of which have no clinical or scientific basis. In some cases they may even be harmful, as they can contain toxic substances or may interact with medicines prescribed by your doctor. It is therefore important that you seek advice from your doctor before embarking on any alternative therapy. Much more research is needed to provide better evidence that various foods, plant extracts and supplements are truly as safe and effective as the manufacturers would have us believe.

7

Prostate awareness

The prostate is a walnut-sized gland that is present only in
men. It is located deep in the pelvis, at the exit of the bladder,
and surrounds the tube known as the urethra (through which
urine flows from the bladder to the outside of the body).
Tiny at birth and throughout childhood, the prostate enlarges
after puberty, stimulated by rising levels of the male hormone
testosterone secreted by the testes, to a volume of around 20 cc.
Although the prostate is small compared with other organs, it
looms ever larger as a potential source of disease and disability
once a man passes middle age.

The prostate is subdivided into three zones: central, transition
and peripheral, which are shown in the diagram opposite.

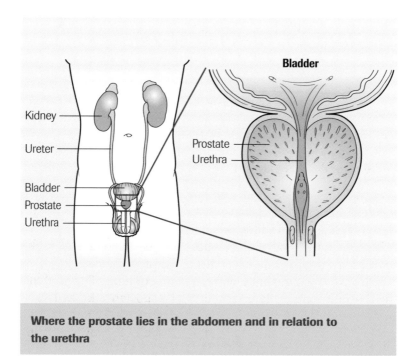

**Where the prostate lies in the abdomen and in relation to
the urethra**

www.prostate-research.org.uk

The peripheral zone is located at the back of the prostate and is the part most susceptible to both prostate cancer and prostatitis. The third and most common prostate problem – benign prostatic hyperplasia (BPH) – develops in the transition zone, which lies in the middle of the gland and surrounds the urethra.

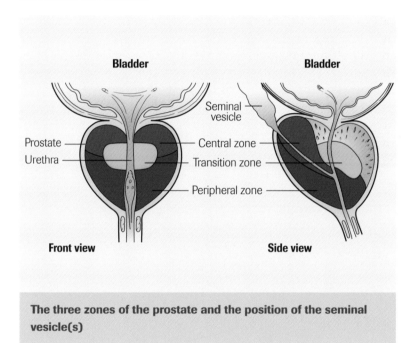

The three zones of the prostate and the position of the seminal vesicle(s)

Function of the prostate

The prostate gland manufactures an important liquefying component of semen. Sperm are produced in the testicles and then stored just behind the prostate in the seminal vesicles. Here, and at the time of ejaculation, the sperm are in a jelly-like medium. At orgasm and ejaculation, the prostate and seminal vesicles contract, mixing their respective contents. The fluid in the prostate contains large amounts of a substance known as prostate-specific antigen (PSA), which liquefies the previously gelatinous sperm mixture, allowing the sperm to move freely in search of an ovum to fertilize.

9

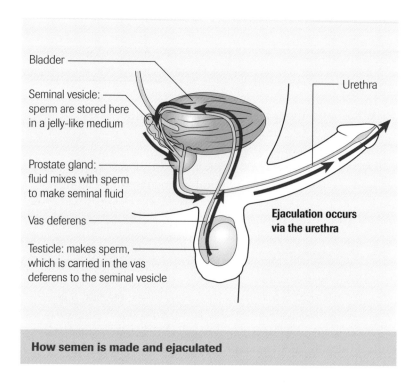

Bladder

Seminal vesicle: sperm are stored here in a jelly-like medium

Urethra

Prostate gland: fluid mixes with sperm to make seminal fluid

Vas deferens

Ejaculation occurs via the urethra

Testicle: makes sperm, which is carried in the vas deferens to the seminal vesicle

How semen is made and ejaculated

Common diseases involving the prostate

Because the prostate surrounds the urethra, any disease of the gland is likely to cause disturbances in urinary flow, and in the frequency and efficiency with which the bladder is emptied. There are three common diseases that may affect the prostate:

- BPH, which results in frequent urination and a reduced urinary stream, and affects almost 50% of men beyond middle age
- prostate cancer, which is now the most common malignancy in men with a 1 in 14 lifetime risk, rising to 1 in 11 for men over 50 years of age
- prostatitis, an inflammatory disease affecting about 1 in 15 mainly younger and middle-aged men, which is characterized by symptoms of pain and discomfort around the anus, scrotum and the area in between (the perineum).

So when should you see your doctor?

Problems with urinating are the most common symptoms of prostate disease. You should visit your doctor if you regularly experience one of the following:

- a weak, sometimes intermittent flow of urine
- difficulty starting to urinate
- a need to urinate frequently
- a need to urinate urgently (you do not feel able to put it off)
- having to go to the toilet several times during the night
- a feeling that your bladder is not completely empty after you have finished urinating
- pain or burning when passing urine
- blood in your urine.

Of course, problems may develop before any symptoms arise. For this reason, it is generally advisable for most men over 50 to have an annual health check, which often includes an assessment of the prostate, including a PSA test. Remember, while a one-off PSA check provides a certain amount of information, regular checks are more informative because they show the rate of the rise in PSA (sometimes called the 'PSA kinetics'). A sudden rise in PSA is rather like a flashing light on the dashboard of your car; it tells you that something is amiss, which, if responded to, will help to prevent eventual breakdown.

The PSA test

PSA, prostate-specific antigen, is a protein-like substance that occurs in abundance in the fluid within the prostate. Testing blood samples to determine the amount of PSA (a 'PSA test') is central to the early detection and selection of effective treatment for prostate cancer. Monitoring a man's PSA level

Prostate gland   Blood vessel

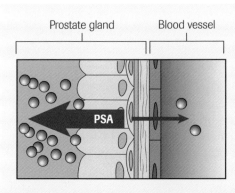

Normal

Cells in the prostate are healthy and organized in a tight pattern. Only a small amount of PSA leaks out of the prostate and gets into the bloodstream

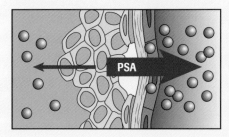

With prostate cancer

Now the cells are disorganized and the layers between the prostate and blood vessel become disrupted. More PSA can leak into the blood vessel as a result

The growth of cancer cells in the prostate disrupts the structure and organization of the tissue. PSA inside the prostate is able to leak into the nearby blood vessels more readily than it does in a healthy prostate. As a result, the amount of PSA in the blood increases, which is why measurement of PSA in a blood sample can help to diagnose prostate cancer

is also extremely helpful once therapy has been started, as it can indicate how effectively treatment is working. If the PSA is rising in spite of treatment, second-line therapies such as oestrogens or chemotherapy with, for example, Taxotere (docetaxel) may be in order.

Basis of the PSA test

Prostate cancer develops from the lining cells of the tiny glands within the prostate whose function is to manufacture PSA. Not surprisingly therefore, prostate cancer cells nearly all continue to secrete PSA. As the cancer grows PSA levels tend to rise. Moreover, as the pre-cancer stage, prostatic intra-epithelial neoplasia (PIN, see page 31) evolves into invasive prostate cancer, the membrane surrounding the prostate may start to break down in small areas. As a consequence, the fluid in the prostate and the PSA it contains start to leak out. The PSA finds its way into the blood and so the amount of PSA in the blood starts to increase. Progressively worsening damage to the prostate makes it more leaky which, in turn, results in higher PSA levels in the blood. A normal PSA level (in a man with no prostate problems) is usually accepted as being below 4 ng/mL (4 nanograms per millilitre), but this rises with age so that in men over 70 a cut-off of 6.5 ng/mL is accepted (see table below). Remember that there is nothing magical about a cut-off value. Recent studies have shown that many men with a PSA below 4 ng/mL may, in fact, harbour small cancers. In younger men, especially, it is the rate

Increase in accepted PSA cut-off with age	
Age	**PSA cut-off**
40–49 years	2.5 ng/mL
50–59 years	3.5 ng/mL
60–69 years	4.5 ng/mL
Over 70 years	6.5 ng/mL

www.prostate-research.org.uk

of the rise in PSA rather than its absolute value that may be important. Current research suggests that a rise of more than 0.75 ng/mL per year may indicate the need for further investigation, although more work is needed to verify this.

PSA in the bloodstream is either free or bound to one of two proteins – antichymotrypsin and alpha macroglobulin. For reasons that are still not clear, in men with prostate cancer the amount of unbound or 'free' PSA is reduced. As a consequence, a reduction in the percentage of free PSA is also an early warning sign for prostate cancer. The cut-off point is usually taken as 18%; values above this indicate benign prostate enlargement, while values less than 18% increase the probability of prostate cancer being present.

When doctors and journalists talk about screening for prostate cancer, they are usually referring to the potential to test every man's PSA level at fixed intervals of time (like the smear test for women), from the age of around 50 onwards. If the test is so useful, why is it not used in this way? There are several points that have to be considered, and the pros and cons of the PSA test are summarized in the table on page 16.

Issues surrounding the PSA test

Overdetection of clinically insignificant cancers

As prostate cancer occurs mainly in men beyond middle age, it is perfectly possible that a small cancer might never grow sufficiently large to cause symptoms during a man's lifetime. The anxiety caused by a 'positive' (high) PSA result might reduce the man's quality of life by causing unnecessary worry, whereas if he remained ignorant of his condition, his life would be unaffected. However, fears of this sort of overdiagnosis of prostate cancer have lessened as doctors increasingly employ 'active surveillance' as a treatment strategy for smaller, less aggressive cancers.

'False-positive' results

An elevated level of PSA in the blood does not necessarily indicate cancer. Indeed, the average PSA level rises with age and any disease of the prostate – particularly BPH, but also prostatitis – can result in an elevated PSA, though usually to a rather minor extent.

A high PSA value, or one that increases over time, will usually prompt a doctor to request a biopsy, which involves taking samples of tissue from the prostate. However, scientific studies have shown that when samples of prostate tissue are examined under the microscope, only one man among four with a PSA value between 4 and 10 ng/mL will be found to have cancer (so three will not have cancer even though their PSA levels are raised).

With a higher cut-off (say PSA above 10 ng/mL), the probability that a subsequent biopsy will confirm prostate cancer rises to more than 60%. Of course, the problem with using a higher cut-off to determine who should receive a biopsy is that as the cut-off value increases, so does the 'false-negative' rate. (False negatives are PSA test results below the cut-off value, but prostate cancer is present; this is illustrated in the diagram on page 17. Remember that early prostate cancer can be present even when the PSA value is below 4 ng/mL.) Also, if cancer is to be identified at a stage when it is still curable, then it should be detected before the PSA rises much above 10 ng/mL.

Recently there has been great interest in measuring the rate of PSA change over time. Although the information on this subject is only provisional, as already mentioned, it seems that men whose PSA rises by more than 0.75 ng/mL per year are at higher risk of harbouring the more aggressive (so-called 'tiger') form of prostate cancer as opposed to a more innocuous 'pussy-cat' tumour, which in fact carries little risk of spread. In order to detect the rate of PSA change, regular (usually yearly) blood tests are required. These can usefully be combined with cholesterol and lipid measurements, provided that fasting blood samples are obtained.

Anxiety before the results become available
The speed with which you get your test results depends on where you have your test. It can take anything from a couple of

The pros and cons of PSA testing

Pros

- Allows early detection of potentially curable prostate cancer

- Permits the doctor to estimate prostate size in a patient with BPH

- Helps the doctor predict response to certain drugs

- Allows the doctor to estimate how advanced the cancer is at diagnosis

- Can be used to monitor men at increased risk of prostate cancer, such as those with a family history

- Can help the doctor estimate the patient's risk of developing prostate cancer in the future

- A negative result is reassuring

- Sequential values provide extra information about cancer risk

- Helpful for monitoring response to treatment

Cons

- Clinically insignificant cancers may be detected causing needless worry and further medical procedures for the patient

- Men without cancer may have a false-positive result (particularly those with borderline PSA values)

- A false-negative result may provide unwarranted reassurance

- There are cost implications – not only regarding the PSA test, but of biopsy and treatment options if the biopsy is positive

- Those undergoing biopsy are exposed to the risks of bleeding and infection

hours to several weeks – obviously those at the longer end of the scale have more opportunity for anxiety. Ask your doctor about the usual waiting time for results in his clinic. However, bear in mind that the most important factor is obtaining an accurate result.

The ideal blood test for prostate cancer

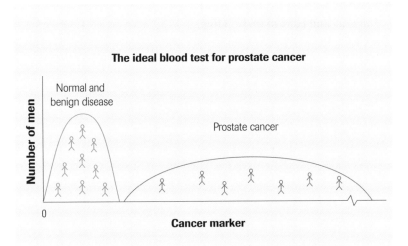

Cancer marker

The present test: prostate-specific antigen (PSA)

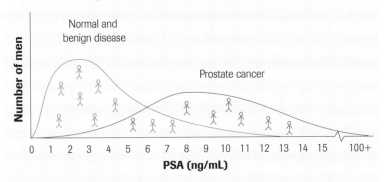

An 'ideal' blood test for prostate cancer should clearly distinguish men who have cancer from those who do not. Although PSA measurement is a useful test, it is not perfect – if a cut-off of 4 ng/mL is used, there is an overlap between patients with BPH or other diseases and those with prostate cancer. Inevitably, this results in some men worrying unnecessarily that they may have cancer

Over-the-counter PSA tests, which will allow self-testing, are becoming available in chemist shops. Like the whole PSA issue, these home tests are bound to be rather controversial.

Exposure of those undergoing biopsy to the risk of complications

Biopsy (in which 6–12 small pieces of prostate tissue are removed so that they can be examined for signs of prostate cancer, see page 26) may result in minor bleeding and the appearance of blood in the semen. This usually settles spontaneously after a few weeks. There is also a small risk of infection, but doctors try to minimize this by prescribing antibiotics for you to take before and for several days after the biopsy. If you have had a biopsy and develop symptoms of infection (especially shaking attacks and a high temperature), contact your doctor immediately.

It's not always cancer

It is worth re-emphasizing that a PSA level that is higher than normal does not necessarily mean that you actually have prostate cancer. Conversely, a normal PSA value does not conclusively exclude the presence of the disease. Both BPH and prostatitis can result in elevated PSA levels in the blood, and your doctor will cross-check your PSA result with your symptoms, the result of a digital rectal examination (see page 22) and probably the results from a biopsy to make the diagnosis. If you have a raised PSA, but a negative result on biopsy, your doctor will probably monitor your PSA level over time. Depending on further results, he may suggest that you have another biopsy at a later date. The value of sequential PSA testing lies in its ability to set a baseline. A sudden or progressive rise above this level may act as an early warning of either prostate cancer development or another disease process within the gland. Urinary infection, for example, or sudden retention of urine requiring a catheter, can both cause the PSA level in the blood to rise sharply.

Your choice

In the end, it is up to you whether you have the PSA test or not, and whether you continue with annual or biannual checks. But make sure you base your decision on reliable information, not the latest newspaper, radio or TV article, or some unsubstantiated internet site, and discuss it with your partner.

The Department of Health has recently changed its policy on PSA testing and has agreed that men should be entitled to this test once they have had enough information to make an informed choice (see www.cancerscreening.nhs.uk/prostate/).

In summary, the PSA test is not perfect, and much work is currently being done to come up with something better. For the time being, however, it is the best we have, and if used intelligently can be a valuable early indicator of problems, benign and malignant, that are developing within the prostate.

A raised or rising PSA: what happens next?

Finding a good urologist

If your GP finds that you have a raised or rising PSA level (usually above 4 ng/mL, but in younger men above 2.5 ng/mL), or a reduced percentage of free PSA (less than 18%) you will probably be referred to a urologist – a specialist in disorders affecting the kidney, bladder and prostate in men (and the urinary tract in women). It is important that you feel comfortable with, and confident in, your urologist. You should understand his explanations of procedures and options, and he should be prepared to discuss fully anything that concerns you or your partner. In this day and age, do not simply accept that the 'doctor knows best' – it is your health and peace of mind at stake here, so make sure that you have had all your questions answered before you leave the consultation room. If you or your family are not happy with your urologist, go back to your GP and discuss the matter with him.

Alternatively, you may want to find your own specialist on a private basis. If this is the case, the first thing to do is to check your health insurance, if you have it. Some companies will not cover your expenses unless you have been referred by your GP. Also, you (or your insurers) may want to check the prices of treatment at an early stage. The clinic should provide a price list for you – if they do not, talk directly to the urologist. If you are not happy with your service, talk to the clinic manager or the urologist (or his secretary) directly – you are a prospective customer and they will be unlikely to want to 'lose' you. If you are still not happy, go back to your GP.

If you find it difficult to voice your concerns face-to-face or if you feel that you might forget some things, write a letter or list so that you can make sure that all your points are answered. It may also be useful to take your partner with you to the consultation. Taking a look at some of the websites listed on page 110 may also be helpful, and these days you can find out a lot about the doctor who is treating you from the internet.

Tests

Some measurements will be taken to assess your general health. For example, height, weight and abdominal girth may be measured, as obesity is a risk factor for prostate cancer, diabetes and heart disease. Your blood pressure may also be checked, as early identification of hypertension is important to prevent the development of complications. For similar reasons, blood tests for sugar and cholesterol (see below) may be carried out.

Your urologist may also repeat tests that your GP has already carried out, such as the PSA and percentage free PSA measurements. He may want to check your situation for himself; for some tests it is important that the samples are always sent to the same laboratory for analysis if you are being monitored over a period of time.

Blood tests

The basis of the PSA test was described earlier on pages 13–14. Other tests, such as your fasting blood sugar and cholesterol level, may be used as indicators of your general health and to rule out diabetes or an abnormal lipid profile (e.g. raised cholesterol). They can also be used to estimate the risk of future problems, such as heart disease or stroke.

Urine tests

You may be asked to provide a urine specimen. This could be checked for bacteria, as you may have a urinary tract infection. It may also be tested for the presence of blood. Blood can be found in the urine if prostate cancer has spread into the urethra, which runs through the prostate, so its presence is a clue to the urologist about the nature of your problem. Other important causes of blood in the urine include bladder stones and bladder cancer, so this is a finding that should not be ignored. Urine may also be routinely tested for sugar in order to detect diabetes.

Physical examination and digital rectal examination

The urologist may examine you in general, but will almost certainly perform a digital rectal examination. Undeniably, it is an uncomfortable experience and one that some men dread, but is actually much less uncomfortable than a visit to the dentist. Urologists perform this day in, day out, but if that does not reassure you, just keep thinking about the consequences of ignoring your condition. A few moments of minor discomfort are surely worthwhile.

Your urologist will put on a glove and apply some lubricant jelly to his finger. He will tell you which position to adopt – probably one where you lie on your side with your legs pulled up towards your chest. He will then gently insert his finger into your rectum, passing through the sphincter muscle that keeps the anus closed. He will then feel your prostate, noting its size, shape, firmness and how its surface feels – an enlarged but soft prostate suggests benign enlargement of the gland, while a firm nodule may indicate cancer. The examination is not painful, just uncomfortable. Try to relax until it is over – it literally only lasts a few moments.

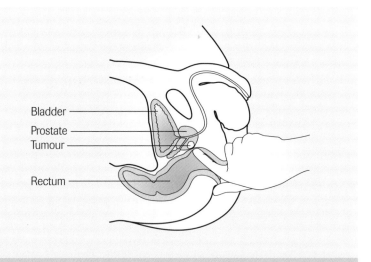

Bladder
Prostate
Tumour

Rectum

A digital rectal examination is uncomfortable but not painful and only lasts a few moments

Urination questionnaire

Prostate cancer may be affecting your ability to empty your bladder or you may have BPH that is affecting your urine flow. In order to investigate your symptoms in a meaningful way, your urologist may give you a questionnaire to fill in (see overleaf). You may be asked to fill it in while you are in the clinic or you may be able to take it home with you to complete and return at your convenience.

If cancer is suspected

If cancer is suspected, your urologist will first need to check whether you do in fact have cancer by performing a biopsy. If you have, he will then need to determine how aggressive it is and how far it has progressed. You may hear a reference to the grade and stage of your cancer. These are important in selecting the best treatment option for you.

Grade

The grade is a measure of how aggressive the cancer is. The cancer cells in the prostate start out looking very similar to normal prostate cells, but start to change their appearance and de-differentiate (i.e. become more aggressive) as the cancer progresses (see page 32). Grading is a means of assessing this process in a standardized way, and is performed in a laboratory by specialized pathologists.

The most common grading system is the Gleason system. From incidental post-mortem findings, we can speculate that grade 1, 'latent' prostate cancer, is probably quite common among men aged over 40; these small tumours often grow very slowly, and so many men will never develop symptoms during their natural lifespan. However, a cancer that progresses more quickly (that is, a more aggressive one) will show a less differentiated pattern, and will be graded higher. The cancerous areas in the prostate may vary and have different grades, so the grades of the two most prominent areas are added together to give a Gleason score (for example, 3 + 4); the maximum is 10 (5 + 5). This figure then gives your doctor an

	Not at all	Less than 1 time in 5	Less than half the time	About half the time	More than half the time	Almost always	Patient score
1 Incomplete emptying Over the past month, how often have you had a sensation of not emptying your bladder completely after you finished urinating?	0	1	2	3	4	5	
2 Frequency Over the past month, how often have you had to urinate again less than 2 hours after you finished urinating?	0	1	2	3	4	5	
3 Intermittency Over the past month, how often have you found you stopped and started again several times when you urinated?	0	1	2	3	4	5	
4 Urgency Over the past month, how often have you found it difficult to postpone urination?	0	1	2	3	4	5	
5 Weak stream Over the past month, how often have you had a weak urinary stream?	0	1	2	3	4	5	
6 Straining Over the past month, how often have you had to push or strain to begin urination?	0	1	2	3	4	5	
7 Nocturia Over the past month, how many times did you most typically get up to urinate from the time you went to bed at night until the time you got up in the morning?	0	1	2	3	4	5+	
Total score							

	Delighted	Pleased	Mostly satisfied	Mixed	Mostly dissatisfied	Unhappy	Terrible
Quality of life due to urinary symptoms If you were to spend the rest of your life with your urinary condition the way it is now, how would you feel about that?	0	1	2	3	4	5	6

A sample questionnaire on urinary symptoms

Gleason score and the risk of prostate cancer progressing

Gleason score	Risk
2–4	Low
5–7	Medium
8–10	High

idea of how quickly your cancer is likely to progress and therefore helps him advise you about treatment.

Stage

The cancer can also be classified according to how far it has spread, that is its 'stage'. The tumour–nodes–metastases (TNM) system is commonly used, and involves the doctor assessing how far your cancer (tumour) has spread in and around the prostate, whether it has spread to the nearby lymph nodes (nodes) and then whether it has spread (metastasized) to the distant lymph nodes and bones. Knowing the stage of your cancer helps you, your family and your urologist to decide on the most appropriate course of action.

Grading and staging tests

PSA measurement and digital rectal examination are both important for staging cancer, but you will almost certainly have to undergo some further tests.

Ultrasound

Ultrasound may be used to assess the size and texture of the prostate; the specific technique is called transrectal ultrasonography (or TRUS for short). A lubricated probe is inserted into the rectum, where it passes high-frequency sound waves through the prostate. Computer analysis of the echoes, which vary according to the density of the tissues the waves are passing through, produces an image of the prostate that can then be seen on a screen. Ultrasound is a relatively simple and safe procedure that is not too uncomfortable, but without a biopsy it cannot be used to tell definitively whether or not cancer is present.

Ultrasound-guided biopsy

Ultrasound-guided biopsy is used to obtain tiny samples of tissue from your prostate that can then be sent to the pathology laboratory for analysis under a microscope. The pathologist can check whether cancer is present and, if it is, grade it. You will probably be recommended for biopsy, an outpatient procedure, on the basis of your PSA level.

Using ultrasound for guidance, a fine, automated needle is inserted into the back passage until it reaches the prostate (shown in the diagram on the previous page). The test is not too painful (not much worse than a visit to the dentist), but you may feel a sharp needle prick as 6–12 tissue samples are taken, even if a local anaesthetic has been used. The results should be available within a few days. Remember, though, that biopsies of the prostate are only tiny samples of the whole gland, so small cancers may sometimes be missed. If the PSA continues to rise in spite of a negative biopsy result a further set of biopsies may be required. Several studies have shown that after 3 sets of negative biopsies prostate cancer is unusual because the rise in PSA that triggered the biopsy is usually the result of benign prostatic hyperplasia (BPH).

You will usually be given antibiotics (tablets or an injection) for 24 hours or immediately before the procedure, and you will be told to continue taking the prescribed antibiotic tablets for several days afterwards. For several weeks after the procedure, you may notice blood in your urine, semen and/or bowel motions. This is quite normal, but if you have any worries, consult your doctor. Urinary infections can occasionally occur as a consequence of the biopsy – if you feel a burning sensation on urination, notice that your urine is cloudy and/or smelly, find that you have to urinate more frequently than normal and/or you develop a temperature, have shaking attacks and feel generally unwell, contact your doctor. He will probably

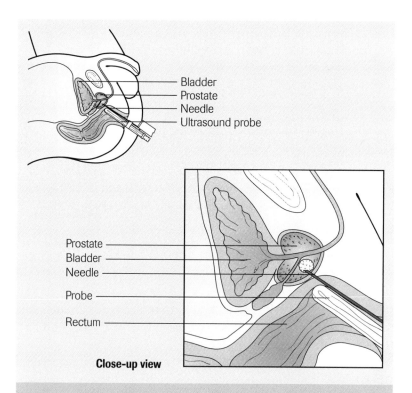

Bladder
Prostate
Needle
Ultrasound probe

Prostate
Bladder
Needle
Probe
Rectum

Close-up view

When a prostate biopsy is performed, a lubricated ultrasound probe is inserted into the rectum to give an accurate view of the prostate. Samples of tissue (usually 6–12) are collected using a fine, automated needle

prescribe more antibiotics or, occasionally, admit you to hospital for treatment using an intravenous drip.

There is no evidence that biopsies cause prostate cancer to spread. The ability to spread (to metastasize) to other parts of the body, such as the skeleton, depends on the characteristics of the cancer cells themselves and tends to occur quite late in the disease.

Bone scans
Bone scans are a means of checking whether the cancer has spread (metastasized) around the body. Two to three hours

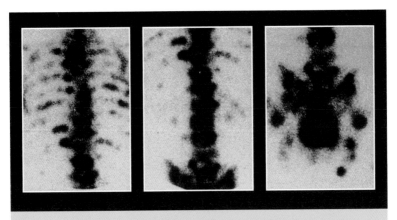

Bone scans from a man with prostate cancer. The dark spots show the presence of secondary cancer in the bones

before you have the scan, a mixture containing radioactive particles (radionuclides) will be injected into your arm. The particles then spread around your body; their pattern, which shows up on the scanner, can reveal 'hot spots', which are dark areas of abnormal blood flow – a sign that cancer may be present. Remember that 'hot spots' can be the result of other diseases, such as arthritis in the joints and spine, so further testing may be necessary to clarify the cause of an abnormal scan. Do not be concerned about the use of radiation here – the amount is so low that the risk to your health is negligible.

MRI

MRI, or magnetic resonance imaging, is a technique whereby a strong magnetic field and radio signals are used to examine sequential cross-sections of the body. The images that result are highly detailed – the urologist can use them to assess the extent of the cancer in the prostate and to check whether any secondary tumours have formed in other regions. The procedure is completely painless, but some people find being in the scanner a little claustrophobic. The results should be available within a few days.

If you have any metal implants, such as a pacemaker or coronary artery stents, it may not be possible to perform an MRI scan, so a CT scan will probably be arranged.

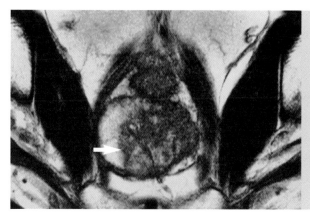

An MRI scan showing cancer (arrowed) in the prostate

CT scanning

CT, or computerized tomography, is similar to MRI in that the technique produces images of sequential slices through the body, but it uses X-rays to build up the images. CT scanning is not as accurate as MRI, but is much less claustrophobic. Occasionally, CT scanning is used to guide biopsy needles to obtain tissue samples from enlarged lymph nodes or other soft tissues. It also helps when planning radiotherapy treatment fields.

Why scans are not always necessary

Although you might think that every man who has been diagnosed with prostate cancer requires scanning, in fact, in men with a PSA below 10 ng/mL, the chances of a positive scan are so low that they are generally not recommended. Many patients feel reassured to know that their scans are clear, but remember that bone scans can give false-positive results and MRI scans can also sometimes be misleading as they cannot reliably detect microscopic spread outside the prostate.

Partin's tables

Although the tests described above seem very 'high tech' and sophisticated, unfortunately they do not always give a very precise answer to the question 'has the cancer spread beyond the gland?' In fact the so-called 'Partin's tables', which compare the findings of the rectal examination, the PSA level

29

and the Gleason score, are still the best way of estimating the risk of spread beyond the prostate capsule.

These tables were developed by Dr Alan Partin, now the Professor of Urology at Johns Hopkins University Hospital, Baltimore, USA. He has shown that the smaller the cancer feels on rectal examination, and the lower the PSA level and Gleason score, the greater the likelihood that the cancer can be completely removed by surgery. These tables can therefore be useful in helping the doctor, patient and family decide together on the best treatment option.

Receiving bad news

Of course, being told that you are suffering from prostate cancer will come as a major shock. In an instant your usually optimistic prospects for the future are transformed. The blow can be lessened, however, if the news is broken sensitively and sympathetically, in the presence of your partner or a close friend, by a caring and informed professional who gives you as much time as you need.

Often nowadays, the consultation with the doctor who delivers the news about the biopsy results is followed immediately by an interview with a urology nurse specialist. This specialist nurse will help to answer any further questions you might have and provide written material about the disease and its treatment. This can be invaluable, because many patients retain only a fraction of the information they are given after the shocking news of a cancer diagnosis. The specialist nurse will also provide details of sources of support from charities, such as the Prostate Research Campaign UK and Cancerbackup, as well as details of patient support groups. (You can find details of sources of further information and support on page 110.)

Although the news may not be what you had hoped for, remember that the outlook for men with prostate cancer is now generally good and, with all the current research effort, is improving all the time.

Prostate cancer – what it is and what causes it

Prostate cancer develops as a result of a progressive series of faults occurring in the genes that control cell growth in the prostate. These faults can be inherited or develop as a result of damage to the DNA, the material that controls the function of the cell, caused by dietary components, cancer-inducing chemicals or radiation. Normally, cells divide only when the body needs them to, and the process is under strict genetic control. When this genetic control breaks down and the cells begin dividing in an unregulated manner, a mass of excess cells forms (a tumour). A tumour can be benign or malignant, depending on its capacity to invade healthy surrounding tissue (if it can invade, it is cancerous). Because of its capacity to invade surrounding areas, cancer can spread to sites around the prostate, in which case it is said to be locally advanced. It can also spread to distant sites in a process known as metastasis, which occurs as the cancer becomes more advanced. Cancer cells can break off from the tumour in the prostate and enter the bloodstream and lymphatic system (the latter is a network of tiny vessels that drain fluid from all the organs in the body). In this way, cancer cells are transported to other parts of the body (for example, the lymph nodes or bones) and, like seeds growing in fertile soil, secondary tumours develop.

Stages of cancer

The earliest stage in uncontrolled cell growth is not actual malignancy, but pre-malignancy, known as prostatic intraepithelial neoplasia (PIN for short). PIN is characterized by a 'heaping up' of cells within the prostate, but there is no invasion of healthy tissue at this stage. With time, however, these dividing cells may develop the ability to invade and occupy the prostate tissue. Such early signs of invasion give

31

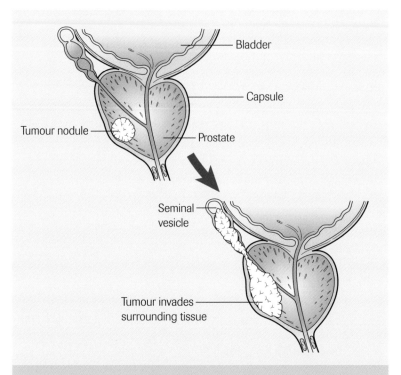

Bladder

Capsule

Tumour nodule

Prostate

Seminal vesicle

Tumour invades surrounding tissue

As prostate cancer develops, it forms a nodule that can then grow and spread to the seminal vesicles and other local structures

the pathologist examining a sample (biopsy) of prostate tissue under a microscope the clue that actual cancer has developed from the pre-malignant PIN changes. At this stage, the level of a substance known as PSA (see page 12) in the blood usually begins to rise – another clue that invasive prostate cancer is developing.

As cancer develops from prostate cells, when looked at under the microscope, early, less aggressive cancers bear a close resemblance to normal tissue. As the cancer becomes more aggressive and potentially dangerous, these similarities are progressively lost. This process is known as 'de-differentiation' and was described in the 1960s by the pathologist Dr Gleason. A sample of prostate tissue is given a 'Gleason grade' according to the shape, size and structure of the cells in the sample. The grading runs from 1 to 5; the higher the number, the more aggressive the cancer (see page 23). Because the cells will not appear uniform across the tissue sample, the two most prominent regions are usually assessed, and the two grades added together to give what is known as the 'Gleason score'. Doctors can use this to estimate the likely outcome for their patients. The higher the score (from 2–10), the more potentially dangerous the cancer in terms of progression.

Once prostate cancer cells have developed the ability to invade tissue, they initially spread locally within the gland and then start to invade the capsule that surrounds the gland. Small tumours can be detected only by examining a biopsy of an apparently normal gland under the microscope; larger cancers can usually be felt by the doctor as a firm nodule during an examination via the back passage (rectum), known as the digital rectal examination.

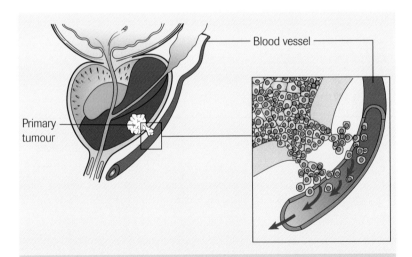

Primary tumour

Blood vessel

As the cancer becomes more advanced, the cells are able to break off from what is known as the primary tumour. These cells enter the blood or lymphatic system, and are transported to distant parts of the body. Once deposited at a site, the cancer cells start to grow and multiply, and new secondary cancers called metastases are formed

At first, the cancer spreads locally to tissues around the prostate, such as the seminal vesicles. Eventually, however, it can spread to more distant sites, such as the bones. The mechanisms by which cancer cells acquire the life-threatening ability to spread (metastasize) are currently the subject of intense scrutiny. Central to the process is the ability to obtain a new blood supply to provide oxygen and nutrients to the cancer cells so that they can grow (all cells have these requirements). The development of a new blood supply has been termed 'angiogenesis', and angiogenesis inhibitors, which include the infamous drug thalidomide, as well as newer agents such as angiostatin, provide a very promising new avenue of treatment for prostate cancer; as yet, however, none of these have been approved for clinical use.

Why do some men get prostate cancer and others do not?

Overall, the lifetime risk of a man developing prostate cancer is now around 10%. Your chance of getting prostate cancer depends on your personal risk factors. A risk factor is something that makes you more likely to develop a certain disease; for example, a high cholesterol level in the blood is a well-known risk factor for heart disease.

Risk factors for prostate cancer

- Belonging to an older age group (usually 50+ years)
- Having a close family member who has had prostate cancer
- Having certain racial origins; for example, it is more common among men of Afro-Caribbean origin
- Following certain eating patterns, such as a diet high in saturated fats
- Low exposure to sunlight

The strongest risk factor for prostate cancer is increasing age. The disease rarely occurs in men under 40, but commonly affects men beyond this age. The average loss of life expectancy

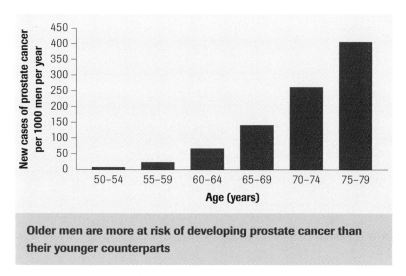

Older men are more at risk of developing prostate cancer than their younger counterparts

is about 9 years – precious retirement years for which most men have been working and eagerly anticipating all their lives.

The next most important risk factor for prostate cancer after age is family history. Like breast cancer, prostate cancer runs in certain families and has been linked to a number of genes. A man whose father, brother, grandfather or uncle has had the disease has an increased risk of developing prostate cancer compared with one without an affected relative. This is particularly the case if the disease developed in the close relative when he was under 60.

Race is also a factor, with men of Afro-Caribbean extraction being at highest risk. These men seem to develop a more aggressive form of the disease and at a younger age than Caucasians. Men of Far Eastern descent seem to be relatively less likely to be affected by the disease.

Can prostate cancer be prevented?

Clearly you cannot change your age, ancestry or race (these are 'non-modifiable risk factors'). However, several other risk factors for prostate cancer have been identified over which you can have some influence – lifestyle factors, such as diet and exercise (see pages 4–5). In addition, various dietary supplements may offer some protection (see pages 5–7).

Geographically, prostate cancer tends to become more common as you move away from the equator; Norway and Sweden have the highest death rates from the disease worldwide. This fact points us to two further possible modifiable risk factors – low vitamin D and low exposure to sunlight, which itself helps the body to produce vitamin D. This evidence provides a good excuse for regular holidays in the sun!

As already mentioned, prostate cancer is characterized by an abnormal overgrowth of prostate cells. As scientists unravel the steps involved in the development of this abnormal cell overgrowth, it is possible, and indeed probable, that we will one day be able to intervene to reverse the earliest phases of the disease. A number of compounds that have this potential are currently being investigated for effectiveness and safety. One of the problems is that it is considerably more difficult (and expensive) to demonstrate that a given drug or vitamin is capable of preventing a disease than it is to show that it can cure a specific problem once it has developed. Because we are never sure exactly who will develop a disease such as prostate cancer, very large numbers of individuals have to be studied for many years (5, 10 or even 15) before we can be certain that a drug can safely and effectively prevent the disease from occurring.

The drug Proscar (finasteride) has been evaluated for its preventative activity. A recent report has revealed that 25% fewer cases of prostate cancer occurred in the men treated with Proscar at a dose of 5 mg/day. Surprisingly though, those cancers that did occur appeared to be more aggressive in nature than those that occurred in the men not treated with Proscar. For this reason, Proscar has not been approved for use as a preventative agent. Another large study, known as REDUCE, is currently looking at a medication that acts in a similar fashion to Proscar, namely Avodart (dutasteride); however, the results are not expected for some time. Recently, reports have begun to appear suggesting that the cholesterol-lowering drugs known as statins, such as Lipitor (atorvastatin), may offer some protection against prostate cancer. This is intriguing, but needs to be verified.

Other so-called chemopreventative agents will doubtless emerge as more research is undertaken.

Case study

Kenneth, a moderately overweight 64-year-old university lecturer, requested a PSA check from his GP after reading about prostate cancer in the newspaper. The result came back a little raised at 5.6 ng/mL. He was referred to his local urologist who rechecked the PSA and examined his prostate, which was found to be enlarged but soft with no nodules. An eight-core biopsy was performed under antibiotic cover and local anaesthesia, which did produce some blood in the semen but no other side effects.

The biopsy revealed the presence of prostatic intraepithelial neoplasia (PIN), a condition regarded as pre-cancerous, in two out of eight cores and some inflammation in several of the remaining cores. No cancer was detected. Ken was advised to initiate lifestyle changes, with an improved diet and more exercise, and to take vitamin E and selenium on a regular basis. He will be followed up and a rebiopsy considered if the PSA rises or if the consistency of the prostate begins to feel suspicious.

Treatment options for prostate cancer that has not spread beyond the gland

The most appropriate treatment for you will depend on several factors:

- how aggressive and advanced your cancer is (the grade and stage)
- your age
- your general health
- you and your family's own informed treatment preferences.

For example, for older men with small tumours and those with other severe illnesses, often the best option is what is known as active surveillance or 'watchful waiting'.

Active surveillance

When you first hear of active surveillance (watchful waiting), you may think 'What a cop-out', and media reports of older patients receiving second-rate healthcare may spring to mind. But active surveillance is not a second-rate option at all – it is often a way of allowing you to retain maximum quality of life.

The chance that a small, slow-growing tumour will cause problems to an older man before the end of his natural life is often relatively slight. On balance, the side effects of the other treatment options would probably cause far greater distress. As the name suggests, although you will not receive treatment, you will have regular check-ups and your urologist will monitor your condition closely with PSA measurements, scans and sometimes repeat prostate scans and biopsies.

If you choose the active surveillance option you must, for your own peace of mind, be convinced that it is right for you. Despite all the progress made in early diagnosis and treatments, a diagnosis of cancer of any kind is still distressing for the patient, and for his family and friends. It would be a rare person who, having been told that he has cancer, then manages to put the diagnosis out of his mind. It is all too easy to understand everything and feel confident that you are doing the right thing while you are in the urologist's consulting room, and then a few weeks later start to feel panicked and uneasy that nothing is being done about your condition. Remember that the whole point of active surveillance is that your quality of life remains good – if you start to worry needlessly, perhaps losing sleep, then your quality of life is suffering. If this happens, pick up the phone or write to your GP or urologist and tell him how you feel. You might also find that becoming involved with a support group helps (see page 114).

Radiotherapy

Radiotherapy is most appropriate for the older man whose cancer is confined to the prostate or thereabouts. But it is also suitable for the younger man whose general health precludes major surgery or in men who are worried about the side effects of surgery. With this type of treatment, radiation is applied to the affected area – the prostate and surrounding tissues – to destroy the cancer cells, leaving normal cells relatively unaffected. You may be offered one of two types of radiotherapy: external-beam radiotherapy is the most commonly used, but another method, called brachytherapy (see page 41), is also becoming more widely available.

External-beam radiotherapy

As the name suggests, a beam of radiation generated by an external source is directed at your lower abdomen. This is normally an outpatient procedure, and the most usual pattern is 20–30 minutes of treatment, 5 days a week for 6–7 weeks.

About 3 months before the radiotherapy, you may be given hormone therapy (see pages 55 and 56). This shrinks the prostate tumour so that the radiation is more likely to destroy the cancer cells, which are now concentrated in a smaller area.

Recently, a new form of radiotherapy – conformal radiotherapy (CFRT) – has been introduced. The use of a so-called 'multi-leaf collimator' allows more accurate targeting of

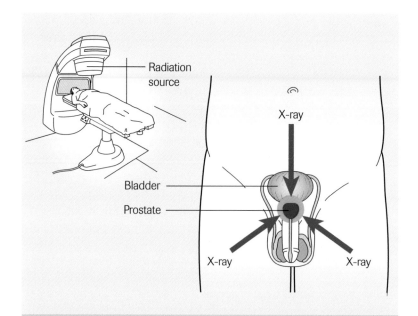

With external-beam radiotherapy, X-rays are produced by an external radiation source and focused on the prostate from three directions

the cancer and so carries a lower risk of side effects – ask your radiotherapist whether it is available in your area. The very latest form of radiation treatment is intensity-modulated radiotherapy (IMRT), which allows high doses of radiation to be precisely shaped to the individual patient's prostate. This very expensive, high-technology equipment is likely to become increasingly available over the next few years.

Possible side effects and risks. The main side effects are bladder irritation and a need to urinate more often. Usually these effects are mild, though a very small proportion of men will be severely affected. You may also feel irritation or discomfort around the rectum, and notice some diarrhoea and bleeding; these effects are usually temporary, lasting only for a few weeks, but may persist for a longer time in some men. Recently, it has been reported that men who have undergone pelvic irradiation for prostate cancer have a slightly higher risk of developing rectal cancer, so you should see your doctor if you have any bleeding from the back passage some time after treatment.

A proportion of men who have undergone radiotherapy will become impotent as a result. This problem tends to develop gradually over 6–12 months, and can usually be overcome with the use of treatments such as Viagra (sildenafil), Cialis (tadalafil) or Levitra (vardenafil) or prostaglandin injections.

Brachytherapy
Brachytherapy has become popular in the USA and is becoming available at an increasing number of centres in the UK. It involves the implantation of radioactive pellets into the

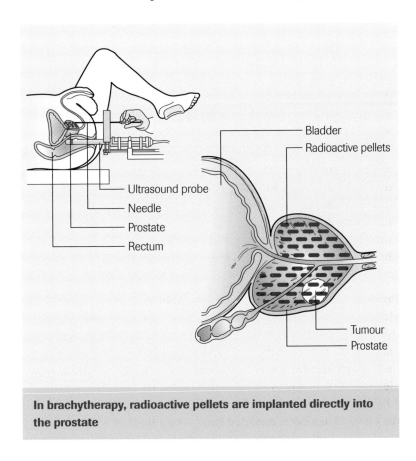

Bladder
Radioactive pellets
Ultrasound probe
Needle
Prostate
Rectum
Tumour
Prostate

In brachytherapy, radioactive pellets are implanted directly into the prostate

prostate, so the radiation is emitted from inside rather than from an external source (as is the case with external-beam radiotherapy). The pellets are left inside the patient where they gradually lose their radioactivity over the following 12 months.

Before the pellets are implanted, the radiotherapist will need to assess your prostate exactly. In order to do so, an ultrasound probe will be inserted into your rectum so that an ultrasound scan can be seen on a computer screen. The pellets – usually between 60 and 100 – are then put into your prostate using needles inserted under anaesthetic through the skin between your scrotum and rectum. You will usually be given a catheter to help you pass urine after the operation, which will have to stay in place for 12 hours or so, but you can normally go home within 24 hours. After brachytherapy the PSA levels gradually decline, but not usually to as low a value as after surgery.

Brachytherapy is most suitable for patients with smaller, lower risk cancers and for men who have small or medium-sized prostates. If TURP has been performed previously to treat BPH, the radioactive seeds cannot be sited correctly in the gland. Pre-treatment with prostate-shrinking drugs, such as LHRH (luteinizing hormone releasing hormone) analogues, can sometimes make brachytherapy suitable for men with

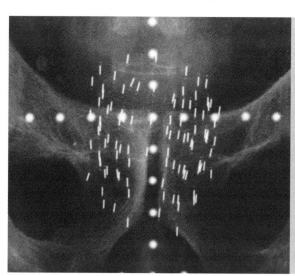

An X-ray showing the radioactive pellets in place in the prostate. The larger dots in the shape of a cross are used to help target the prostate

especially large glands. Brachytherapy is not appropriate for men whose cancer has spread beyond the prostate.

Possible side effects and risks. Up to 10 years after treatment, the results appear to be good in terms of keeping the PSA level down and local cancer control. As the radiation is being targeted at the prostate so accurately, urinary problems and rectal damage are probably less common after brachytherapy than after external-beam radiotherapy. Problems with potency, though, are still common. Only time will tell just how effective it is.

Radical prostatectomy

A radical prostatectomy is a surgical procedure in which the prostate, seminal vesicles and a sample of some nearby lymph nodes are removed. It is a technically difficult operation and, as a result, is usually carried out only in certain hospitals by surgeons with particular expertise and experience. Because it is a fairly major operation, and pelvic surgery (whether open or laparoscopic) always carries certain risks, a radical prostatectomy is most suitable for otherwise healthy, younger men (generally those under 70) whose cancer appears not to have spread to the distant lymph nodes or bones.

The open operation is carried out under a general anaesthetic, and usually takes 1–3 hours; you should expect to stay in hospital for 4–7 days. An 8–10 cm lateral or vertical cut will be made through your abdomen above the pubic bone (or less commonly through the perineum), and your prostate and seminal vesicles will be removed. Samples from the lymph nodes nearest to your prostate will also be taken to check whether the cancer has spread. The so-called cavernous nerves, which lie close to the prostate and are important for achieving an erection, will be identified and the surgeon will take particular care not to disturb them (this may not be possible if the cancer has spread very close to the nerves); this is called a nerve-sparing approach. A catheter will be inserted into the penis so that urination can continue while the join (technically called the anastomosis) between the bladder and

43

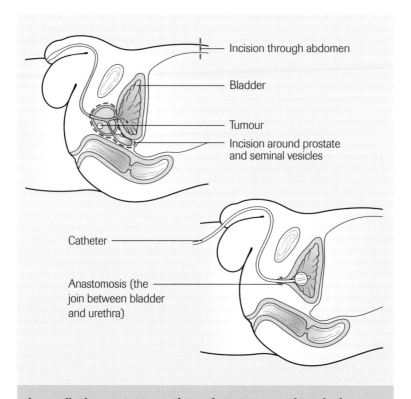

Incision through abdomen

Bladder

Tumour

Incision around prostate
and seminal vesicles

Catheter

Anastomosis (the
join between bladder
and urethra)

In a radical prostatectomy, the entire prostate and seminal vesicles are removed through an incision in the abdomen. Sometimes nearby lymph glands are also removed. The urethra is joined to the bladder and a catheter is inserted to drain urine

urethra heals. The catheter will usually have to stay in place for up to a fortnight (so you will often have to keep it for a week or so after you go home). The scar from the operation heals quite quickly and after a few months will be almost invisible.

You will need to take it easy when you return home from hospital; the usual period of convalescence is 6–8 weeks, but you may still feel tired even after this time. Avoid lifting heavy objects for several months. Some guidelines as to what you should and should not do after the operation are shown in the table opposite.

After a radical prostatectomy

Returning to work

- Possible after 6–8 weeks

- A longer period of absence will be necessary if your job involves heavy lifting

- Your doctor will give you a sick note

Driving

- Do not drive for 2–4 weeks after the operation

Sexual activity

- Do not attempt to have sex for 6–8 weeks

- After this time, you can get back to normal. Orgasm can usually be reached, but there will be no ejaculate and your erection will be weak initially

Drinking

- Try to drink more (non-alcoholic drinks) than you would do normally. The resulting increase in the volume of urine produced can help protect against infection

- You can drink alcohol (but, of course, for your general health, this should be in moderation)

Exercise

- Rest as much as possible for the first 2 weeks

- Avoid any heavy work, such as lifting, carrying or digging, for several months

- Sports and exercise can be resumed after about 1 month, but be guided by how you feel and start off very gently (swimming is a good exercise to begin with)

Laparoscopic and robotic radical prostatectomy

Recent technological developments have enabled the prostate to be removed using telescopes and 4–6 small incisions ('minimally invasive surgery'). The advantages of this technique include reduced blood loss and a quicker recovery time, but the disadvantages are a longer operating time and the difficulty in training surgeons to perform what is a technically very demanding procedure. After puncturing the abdominal wall, the abdominal cavity is distended with gas (carbon dioxide) and the operation performed by the surgeon who is guided by the magnified image on a television monitor.

The very latest development is the use of the da Vinci robot to assist with the laparoscopic operation. This device, which costs around £1.5 million, allows three-dimensional visualization at 10 times magnification and very precise control of movement, which may reduce blood loss and enable better preservation of the nerve bundles that are important for

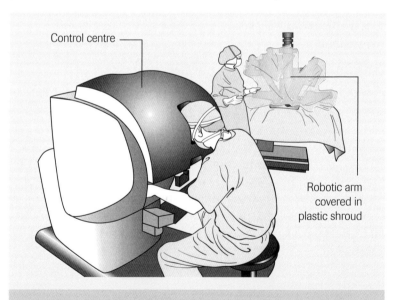

Control centre

Robotic arm covered in plastic shroud

The da Vinci robot enables very precise control of movement, which can help to preserve the nerves that lie close to the prostate and are important for sexual function

erections. The American surgeons who originally developed the technique recently reported that more than 80% of their patients were able to have satisfactory intercourse some months after surgery. At the time of writing, there are over 250 robots in action in the USA, but only a handful in the UK, though this number is likely to increase as results seem good.

PSA level after surgery

After the operation, your PSA level will be checked every 3 months for at least a year. It should drop to about 0.2 ng/mL soon after the operation and then gradually reduce further, ideally to below 0.1 ng/mL, but this will depend to some extent on the laboratory that analyses the sample; some laboratories have machines that only measure PSA as low as 0.5 ng/mL, whereas others have machines that can measure as low as 0.1 or even 0.01 ng/mL.

If your PSA starts to rise because the cancer has not been completely removed (remember that almost all prostate cancer cells manufacture and secrete PSA), you will usually need further treatment.

When further treatment is needed

In between one-tenth to one-third of all men who undergo radical prostatectomy, the cancer will be found to have spread to the margin of the prostate once the pathology report is available. This finding is particularly likely in men whose PSA level is above 10 ng/mL. As a consequence, the operation will sometimes not be 100% successful in these men as the cancer has not been wholly removed from the body. If this is the case for you, your doctor may recommend a 'mop-up' course of radiotherapy or some long-term drug therapy with anti-androgens (see pages 55 and 56).

Possible side effects and risks

A radical prostatectomy, even using the latest laparoscopic and robotic technology, is major surgery and, as such, has side effects that you should consider when deciding whether this is the appropriate course of action for you. For men who may have wanted children, infertility from the surgery needs to be talked through thoroughly with their doctor and partner. Sperm banking is one option that could be considered.

Some men also experience a degree of temporary urinary incontinence after the operation (see page 102). For most, incontinence is mild – a leakage of a small amount of urine on, for example, coughing. A very small proportion of men have severe incontinence requiring further treatment, but very few have a permanent problem, other than having to wear a small pad for security.

Impotence (difficulty achieving an erection) is another side effect and affects many men who have undergone a radical prostatectomy. The risk is reduced where a surgeon uses a nerve-sparing approach but, even so, potency cannot be guaranteed. Although impotence can usually be treated quite effectively, the surgeon should discuss this with you in detail before surgery, and you should discuss it with your partner. Recent evidence suggests that early active rehabilitation using Viagra (sildenafil) or similar agents, such as Levitra (vardenafil), can help to restore sexual function after surgery (see page 104).

Internal scarring from the operation is a further potential complication. If your urine flow deteriorates after surgery, it may mean that you will have to undergo dilatation (stretching) of the join between the bladder and urethra; this is usually curative, but sometimes has to be repeated. Some patients will require a period of self-catheterization to ensure that the join between the bladder neck and the urethra remains wide open as it heals (see page 103).

On the positive side, for men who have BPH as well as prostate cancer, radical prostatectomy can potentially offer a 'double cure' as the prostate, the source of the BPH symptoms, is removed.

The risks associated with radical prostatectomy are those that are generally associated with major surgery – blood loss or blood clots, an adverse reaction to the general anaesthetic and infection.

Your chance of experiencing side effects and the likely success of the operation are governed largely by the expertise of your urologist. If you are offered this operation, you should ask your urologist a number of questions.

- How many radical prostatectomies have you performed (more than 100 is a respectable number) and how many in the last year?
- What were the results of these operations, in terms of removing the cancer, and what was the proportion of patients who were free from the major side effects of impotence and incontinence? (More than 50% of patients younger than 60 years of age able to have intercourse and less than 2% of patients with severe incontinence are good results.)
- Will you be performing my surgery personally?
- Will you be there to help if I have postoperative problems?
- When will the pathology report be available?
- How often will I be seen for follow-up?
- Will I be given help with sexual rehabilitation?

Surgery or radiotherapy?

Ultimately, when you have weighed up the pros and cons with your urologist, the choice will be yours and that of your immediate family. The risks associated with radical prostatectomy or radiotherapy and a summary of the pros and cons of each are shown in the tables below and overleaf.

Risks associated with radical prostatectomy and radiotherapy			
	Men who die as a result	Men who become impotent as a result	Men who suffer mild to severe incontinence
External-beam radiotherapy	Less than 0.1%	30–50%	1–2%
Brachytherapy	Less than 0.1%	30–50%	2%
Radical prostatectomy	0.6%	30–70%	2–15%

The pros and cons of radical prostatectomy versus radiotherapy

Radical prostatectomy

Pros

- Offers a cure for tumours confined to the prostate
- Allows the doctor to stage your tumour accurately
- Coexisting BPH is treated
- Your PSA level should become undetectably low
- You are likely to feel reassured about your condition after the operation
- Monitoring for cancer reappearance is easy
- Radiotherapy can be given afterwards if the cancer returns

Cons

- Major surgery
- Small risk of severe bleeding associated with operation
- Success/side effects depend on the skill of the urologist
- Possible side effects (see text)

Radiotherapy/brachytherapy

Pros

- Offers a potential cure
- Avoids prolonged catheterization and surgery
- Given on an out-patient or short-stay basis
- Hormone therapy can increase the chance of success

Cons

- Treatment is prolonged (6 weeks in external-beam radiotherapy)
- It is relatively difficult to assess whether the treatment has been successful
- Accurate staging is not possible
- Coexisting BPH is untreated
- You may feel more concerned about the possible chance of success afterwards
- Your PSA level may not drop to very low levels
- Repeat radiation treatment is not possible
- Surgery after radiotherapy carries greater risks and is only suitable for selected cases
- Possible side effects (see text)

How do I make the choice?

Until the results of ongoing studies are available, it will not be known for certain which is the safest and most effective treatment for localized prostate cancer. Until then, there will be a choice of treatments, which the patient must decide for himself. Critical to this choice is the confidence that you feel in your doctor and his team, so it is important to find a good specialist team and weigh up the pros and cons with them, before deciding for yourself which treatment is right for you.

The long-term picture

Long-term studies provide information on the prospects of men who have undergone these procedures. While many men want this kind of information, it is important not to take the figures given here too much to heart without discussing your own individual circumstances with your urologist. Progress in medicine means that patients' long-term prospects are improving all the time, and in due course the results of ongoing clinical studies will resolve many controversies.

Active surveillance

The likelihood that your cancer will spread depends, as has already been said, on the nature of your cancer (that is, how aggressive it is). For men whose cancer has a low Gleason score (i.e. well-differentiated tumours), the 10-year survival rate is 87%, which means that, after 10 years, 87 men in 100 will not have died from prostate cancer. With more aggressive cancers (those with higher Gleason scores), the survival rate drops considerably (the 10-year survival rate for men with poorly differentiated tumours has been put at 26%). Watchful waiting is often a good option to start with as more active treatment can always be instituted if signs of cancer progression develop.

Radical prostatectomy

More than 80% of men who have this operation are alive 10 years afterwards, and 60% are still alive at 15 years. A Scandinavian study compared the long-term outcomes of men

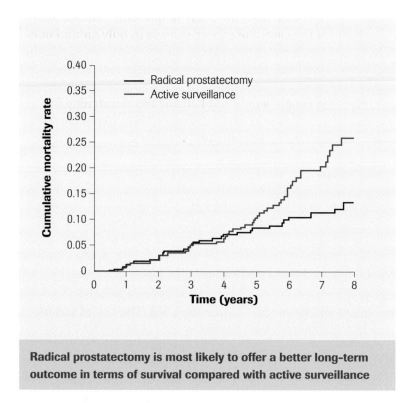

Radical prostatectomy is most likely to offer a better long-term outcome in terms of survival compared with active surveillance

who chose active surveillance with those treated by radical prostatectomy. The results suggest that radical prostatectomy is the treatment option most likely to offer a complete cure for younger men, as it physically removes both the cancer and the entire prostate from the body, making recurrence and spread to the bones much less likely. Another study published recently also showed a survival advantage in patients treated with surgery after 8 years of follow-up.

Results from a study by Pound and colleagues confirm that 82% of men undergoing radical prostatectomy at Johns Hopkins Hospital in Baltimore (USA) were free of recurrence at 15 years (as determined by PSA measurement). The study also offers some comfort to those men whose PSA level rises years after the operation. As we have already said, after a radical prostatectomy, your PSA level drops to an undetectable level and, if it starts rising again, it can signal cancer recurrence. The data from the study in question indicate that, though this is the case, the cancer spreads in only around one-third of men with an elevated PSA. Furthermore, unless a man had a particularly aggressive cancer (in which case his PSA level would tend to rise relatively quickly after the operation), the spreading cancer would not become life-threatening for several years, and would likely be amenable to treatment with radiotherapy or LHRH analogues (see page 56).

Radiotherapy

At best, the survival rates with radiotherapy are comparable to those associated with radical prostatectomy. Several published studies have put the 15-year survival rates at 40–60% (that is, in a group of 100 men, between 40 and 60 will still be alive after 15 years). Recent data suggest that the ongoing use of LHRH injections or anti-androgens to shrink the prostate ahead of radiotherapy can increase the likelihood that treatment will be successful (see page 56). The risk of serious side effects with radiotherapy is decreasing as improved technology means that the cancer-destroying rays can be targeted more accurately at the cancer, leaving adjacent structures, such as the rectum, undamaged. Proponents of brachytherapy also report improving results as techniques and patient selection are enhanced. However, problems with potency are still frequently encountered after radiotherapy and, in fact, are much more common when this treatment is combined with hormone therapy.

A sequential rise in PSA after either external beam radiotherapy or brachytherapy does suggest that recurrence has occurred. Although salvage surgery is technically feasible in some cases, it is often difficult and associated with a high complication rate. Sometimes, cryosurgery or high-intensity focused ultrasound (HIFU) can be used to destroy the residual cancer (see pages 69 and 70), but more commonly hormone therapy is used.

Case study

Douglas, a 58-year-old banker, with an uncle and a father who had both suffered from prostate cancer, went to his GP complaining of the need to get out of bed several times at night to pass urine. A PSA test was requested which came back elevated at 7.8 ng/mL. He was referred to his local urology department and underwent an eight-core biopsy of the prostate, the results of which revealed Gleason grade $4 + 3 = 7$ adenocarcinoma in two cores on the left side of the gland. An MRI scan showed no evidence of disease outside the prostate.

He researched his treatment options on the internet and discussed his case with various helplines. He was attracted to both high-intensity focused ultrasound (HIFU) and brachytherapy as he was nervous about surgery. Further investigations confirmed that his prostate was enlarged and that he was not emptying his bladder properly, and so he followed the advice of his urologist and underwent open radical prostatectomy.

He made a rapid recovery and, on removal of the catheter, was able to pass urine with an improved flow and was completely continent. Examination of the tissue removed confirmed a 2-cm tumour on the left that had been completely excised. Currently, his PSA is undetectable and he is able to function sexually with the help of 100 mg tablets of Viagra.

If prostate cancer has spread or recurs after treatment

Locally advanced disease

If your cancer has spread outside your prostate, but has not yet spread to the lymph nodes close by or to more distant locations, such as the bones, it is described as being 'locally advanced'. (In the TNM staging system, this state is known as T3–N0–M0.) The treatment options for such disease are:

- active surveillance or watchful waiting (for older, less fit men, as before)
- hormone therapy
- intermittent hormone therapy
- hormone therapy followed by radical prostatectomy
- hormone therapy followed by radiotherapy
- anti-androgen alone (monotherapy).

Active surveillance

The rationale behind adopting the approach of active surveillance has been outlined earlier (see pages 38 and 39). However, it is important to realize that at this stage, because the cancer is more advanced, it is likely to cause symptoms and become life-threatening more quickly than a low-grade cancer that is still confined to the prostate. Active surveillance for locally advanced prostate cancer is therefore mainly applicable to older men with a shorter life expectancy.

Hormone therapy

Hormone therapy is sometimes called 'cytoreduction', and has been touched on in the previous section. There are usually two components:

55

- LHRH analogues; LHRH is a naturally occurring hormone, and the 'analogue' part of the name means that it is a synthetic form with a structure similar to the natural form
- anti-androgens, which block the action of the male hormone testosterone in the body.

Testosterone, an androgen or male hormone, is produced in the testicles and has the effect of stimulating cancer growth. The aim of hormone therapy is to reduce the effect of testosterone by switching off testosterone production (the LHRH analogues) and/or by dampening its effects on the cancer (the anti-androgens). The overall effect is that the tumour size is reduced and the progression of the tumour is delayed (hormone therapy does not offer a complete cure, however).

Usually, implants containing a LHRH analogue are inserted by injection at either monthly or 3-monthly intervals. Your body may react to the first injection by initially increasing the amount of testosterone it makes – this is the so-called 'flare' effect. To counter this, you will probably be given an anti-androgen, such as Casodex (bicalutamide), to take a few days before and then continued for several weeks at the beginning of treatment with the LHRH analogue.

Possible side effects. As a consequence of stopping the production of testosterone, men receiving a LHRH analogue lose their sex drive and are unable to achieve an erection. This is gradually reversed if the drug is stopped. Some men also experience hot flushes – these may be eased by low doses (50 mg/day) of Cyprostat (cyproterone acetate).

Anti-androgens may cause mild stomach upsets and diarrhoea. Rarely, they can have a deleterious effect on your liver (so you will need regular blood tests while you are taking these tablets).

How effective is hormone therapy? Hormone therapy alone reduces the tumour size and slows the cancer progression in around 80% of men with locally advanced disease. It does not destroy all the cancer cells, so the cancer is not cured, but its progression is significantly delayed and the effects of other treatments, such as radiotherapy, are enhanced.

Intermittent hormone therapy

Intermittent hormone therapy is a newer approach to hormone therapy. An LHRH analogue is given for about 36 weeks and is then discontinued (providing the PSA level has dropped down to a normal value). When the PSA level returns to a predetermined level, the hormone treatment is started again. Some doctors believe that this might make the cancer cells susceptible to the drug for longer than they would be if treatment was continued without a break. Studies looking at the long-term safety and effectiveness of this approach are under way, but for the moment it is still experimental.

Hormone therapy followed by radical prostatectomy

Some doctors believe that shrinking the tumour with hormone therapy before carrying out a radical prostatectomy increases the chance of removing all the cancer. This approach is being tested in long-term studies. The latest data suggest, however, that there are no concrete, long-term advantages to having hormone treatment before surgery, so this approach is not generally recommended.

Hormone therapy followed by radiotherapy

Again, studies are being carried out to see whether hormone treatment before radiotherapy gives better results than radiotherapy alone. In this case, the results are encouraging, suggesting that the hormone treatment does indeed offer a benefit in terms of curing, or at least delaying, the progress of disease. This is probably because the shrunken tumour is more susceptible to the anti-cancer effects of ionizing radiation. In men at higher risk, the hormone therapy is often continued for several years after the initial treatment.

Anti-androgen monotherapy

There is now scientific evidence that an anti-androgen drug alone (i.e. monotherapy) can also help to slow the progress of advanced cancer, particularly when bone metastases are not present. The advantage of this approach is that anti-androgens have less effect on sex drive and are less likely to cause

57

impotence than the long-acting injectable LHRH analogues. Breast tenderness and enlargement can occur but, although these side effects can be troublesome, they can usually be prevented by a short course of radiotherapy to the nipple areas. Liver function is only rarely disturbed by agents such as Casodex (bicalutamide), but blood testing should be performed to be sure. Worries in Scandinavia about cardiac side effects have not been borne out by studies in other countries, so this treatment is considered by most doctors to be completely safe.

Case study

Andrew, a 73-year-old retired decorator, went to see his GP complaining of difficulty passing urine. His PSA was found to be raised at 11.7 ng/mL and on examination his prostate felt hard and irregular. He was referred to his local urology department, and prostate biopsy as well as bone and MRI scans were arranged. These confirmed a Gleason score of $4 + 4 = 8$ prostate cancer with local spread to the seminal vesicles, but no involvement of either lymph nodes or bones.

Treatment options were discussed and surgery was discounted because of his age and the stage of the cancer. He opted for a course of conformal external beam radiotherapy preceded by 3 months' hormone treatment with Zoladex to reduce the size of the tumour. He tolerated the radiation treatment well, although he did complain of loss of libido and some rectal bleeding towards the end of therapy.

For the 2 years since then his PSA has remained stable and suppressed, and he is being followed up in clinic.

Metastatic disease

Once prostate cancer has spread to the lymph nodes and to distant sites, most frequently the bones, it is referred to as metastatic disease (the metastases are the secondary growths that occur at the distant site); in the TNM staging system, this state is known as T3–N1–M1. This is an advanced form of cancer, and one that is associated with a relatively poor outlook, but there is no need to give up hope.

This stage of cancer can still be treated and progression of the disease can be delayed for several years or sometimes longer. The treatment options are:

- orchidectomy (surgical removal of both testicles)
- hormone therapy with LHRH analogues
- 'maximal androgen blockade', which is hormone therapy with a combination of LHRH analogue and anti-androgen.

Orchidectomy

Orchidectomy is a surgical procedure in which both the testicles are removed. The reasoning behind this is that, as testosterone is produced in the testicles, their removal stops its production altogether. Most men (more than 80%) respond positively to this treatment, with the progression of their cancer slowing markedly for around 18 months and sometimes much longer.

The operation is straightforward and is performed under a local or general anaesthetic in around 30 minutes. In selected patients, silicone testicular prostheses may be inserted to improve the cosmetic result. The scrotal sac is opened and the testicles are snipped out. You may be allowed out of hospital on the same day, although often your surgeon will want you to stay in overnight to check for bruising. You must take things easy for a week or two, and you should also take regular baths or showers to keep the wound clean. Afterwards, the scrotum will look a little bruised, and later somewhat shrivelled and empty, unless prostheses have been used.

Although the operation seems rather drastic, and some men are concerned about 'castration' and the appearance of their scrotum afterwards, it is a one-off procedure and so avoids the need to take a prolonged course of hormone therapy.

Possible side effects and risks. As your body will be unable to produce testosterone after the operation, you will lose your sex drive and be unable to achieve an erection. You will also be infertile. These effects are irreversible, so consider the implications fully before consenting to an orchidectomy. Potential complications of the surgery are relatively few, but

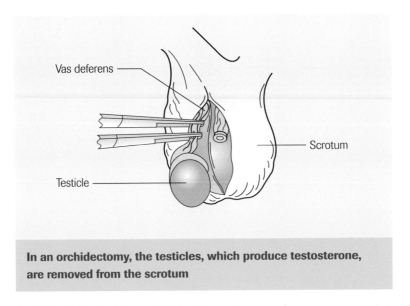

In an orchidectomy, the testicles, which produce testosterone, are removed from the scrotum

bruising, blood clots and infections do occur in some men. Hot flushes may result from the hormone changes in your body. You will not become 'feminized' or find that your voice changes, but you may notice that you lose some body hair and may have to shave rather less often. There is also often a change in skin texture and a theoretical risk of the brittle bone disorder known as osteoporosis.

Hormone therapy

LHRH analogues (see page 56) achieve the same result as removal of the testicles by blocking the production of the male hormone testosterone, and thus reducing the stimulation of cancer growth. LHRH analogues, such as Zoladex (goserelin), are usually administered as an implant, which is injected just under the skin of your abdomen. The procedure is repeated every month or 3 months. As with orchidectomy, a high proportion of men (more than 80%) respond to this treatment and the beneficial effects usually last for around 18–36 months. In terms of effectiveness and safety, there is little to choose between hormone therapy and orchidectomy, but most men prefer the former.

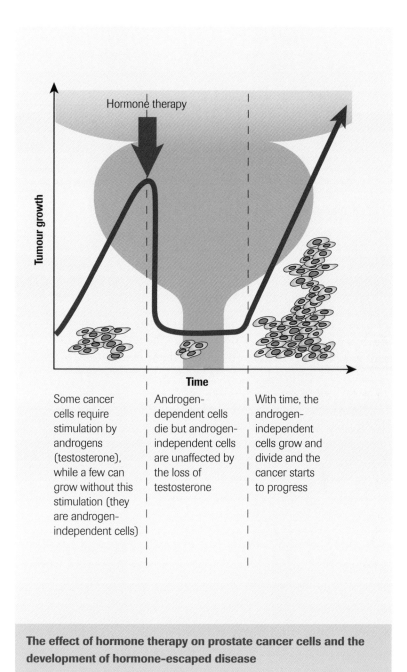

The effect of hormone therapy on prostate cancer cells and the development of hormone-escaped disease

Possible side effects and risks. At first, the LHRH analogue actually increases testosterone production for a few days. Bone pain may increase as a consequence, and urinary symptoms may worsen. This is known as the 'flare' phenomenon. There is even a remote risk of the cancer causing pressure on the spinal cord and thus paralysis. To counter these effects, anti-androgens are usually given for 2 weeks before and then for the first 2–6 weeks of LHRH analogue treatment; these effectively block the effect of testosterone on the cancer.

Maximal androgen blockade

Maximal androgen blockade combines the use of LHRH analogues with long-term anti-androgens. Whether or not this approach is superior to that using LHRH analogues only or orchidectomy is not entirely clear. Some studies show men respond for a longer length of time with this treatment, while others have failed to show such an effect. Many doctors do have confidence in this approach, though, and feel that it is particularly appropriate for younger, relatively fit men with advanced prostate cancer.

Possible side effects. As outlined previously, treatment with LHRH analogues results in a loss of sex drive and impotence. Hot flushes can also be a problem but sometimes respond to treatment with Cyprostat (50 mg/day). The other part of the treatment, anti-androgens, may upset your stomach and can sometimes cause diarrhoea.

Recurrence

Almost inevitably, cancers that initially respond to the above hormonal treatments eventually begin to grow again (the diagram on the previous page explains why this happens). This stage of prostate cancer is often referred to as hormone-relapsed prostate cancer.

If you reach this stage, your doctor may recommend one of the following treatment options:

• modifying existing hormonal therapy by adding or withdrawing anti-androgen

- cytotoxic chemotherapy (drugs that destroy the cancer cells)
- hormone therapy (this is different from that discussed earlier)
- another form of treatment that aims to prevent substances in the body from stimulating further growth of the cancer.

Bisphosphonates

Since prostate cancer frequently spreads to the bone, a class of drugs known as bisphosphonates, which act to stabilize the skeleton and reduce bone loss, may be helpful. A recent study has demonstrated that Zometa (zoledronic acid) administered by intravenous infusion every 3 weeks can delay the development of skeletal problems, such as fracture, by up to 5 months. Side effects of this treatment are relatively minor; some patients develop a flu-like illness during the infusion but this is usually short-lived. More and more men with advanced prostate cancer are now being offered this treatment option, and studies are underway to determine whether bisphosphonates may even prevent metastases in the bone developing in the first place.

Cytotoxic chemotherapy

Cytotoxic chemotherapy is an option, but the drugs used can have unpleasant side effects, such as sickness and hair loss. Increasingly effective chemotherapy drugs are now available, so if your doctor discusses this with you, ask what side effects you might expect and whether it is possible to counter them effectively. Oncologists rather than urologists are experts in this area.

So what is the point of these drugs? It is possible that chemotherapy might give you an extra few months or even years, and if the side effects are minimal or can be overcome, you might feel that this option is worthwhile. New drugs, such as Taxotere (docetaxel), have recently been shown to improve survival rates. Taxotere given every 3 weeks may result in a sharp reduction in PSA values as well as an improvement in quality of life. Side effects include nausea, vomiting, hair loss and a reduction in the white cell count in the blood, known as

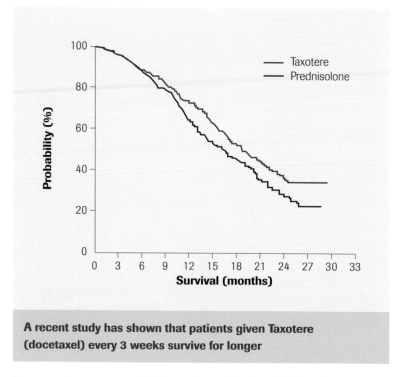

A recent study has shown that patients given Taxotere (docetaxel) every 3 weeks survive for longer

leucopenia – your urologist and oncologist will be able to discuss the latest treatments with you and organize treatment in an oncology centre.

Hormone treatment

Oestrogens, female hormones, may offer some benefit at this stage of your disease. They appear to be able to reduce stimulation of cancer growth and they may also damage the cancer cells directly. The reason that oestrogens are not used in earlier disease is that they can have some potentially serious side effects, such as nausea, blood clots and other cardiovascular complications, such as heart attacks or even strokes. Many doctors advise that you take a low dose of aspirin (75 mg) if you take oestrogen-based drugs to help overcome the potential cardiovascular side effects. Oestrogens should not be used if you have previously had problems with either blood clots or heart failure.

Other treatments

There are a number of what are called 'growth factors' in the body that stimulate the progression of prostate cancer. Blocking the action of these growth factors should potentially block their stimulatory effects on the cancer. However, the drugs that are being developed with this aim are very new and are still under investigation. Angiogenesis inhibitors have already been mentioned (see page 34) and immunotherapy holds some promise. Again though, if you do eventually reach this stage, knowledge of the effects of these drugs may then be such that your doctor is able to prescribe them for you.

Palliative care

Palliative care aims to provide you with support to make you feel comfortable and composed in the final stages of the illness. Over recent years, considerable progress has been made in this area, and medical opinion now holds that no patient need feel the pain or discomfort that was characteristic of the last stages of cancer in bygone years. If your cancer progresses to this stage, you will usually be assigned a palliative care team – specialist doctors and nurses who have considerable expertise and experience in this area, and who will support you and your family. You will have opportunities to talk to members of the team about your care, and you should discuss any medical, social or financial worries that you have.

Patients with very advanced prostate cancer tend to experience bone pain, and you may be given strong and effective painkillers to help overcome this. In addition, you might have radiotherapy (either as a short course or a one off). Another effective method of alleviating bone pain is with injections of a radioactive substance known as strontium. If you are offered radiotherapy, make sure that you know whether it is likely to result in other side effects, such as nausea and vomiting, so that you can weigh up the advantages and disadvantages in the light of all the facts and your own circumstances. In this situation, the first consideration of the medical team should be to preserve your dignity and help your family and friends to support you, ideally in your own home.

Case study

Bill, a 65-year-old retired driver who hails originally from Jamaica, went to see his GP complaining of tiredness, weight loss and low back pain. X-rays of the spine suggested the presence of metastatic cancer and his PSA result came back at 556 ng/mL.

He was referred urgently for prostate biopsy, which revealed a Gleason score of 5 + 4 = 9; a bone scan confirmed multiple metastases particularly involving the spine. Bill was informed of the diagnosis in the presence of his supportive family and agreed to commence androgen ablation (i.e. hormonal) therapy. After 5 days of antiandrogen therapy, a 3-month depot injection of an LHRH analogue was given which quickly relieved his back pain and improved his general health. His PSA also fell quickly to a lowest value of 3.8 ng/mL, but then started to rise. At this point, Bill was referred to his local oncology department, and further blood tests and scans were arranged that confirmed that hormone relapse had occurred. He was treated with 3-weekly infusions of Taxotere (docetaxol) and Zometa (zoledronic acid) with some improvement in his well-being and a substantial fall in his PSA. He remains under follow-up and supported by his family and the palliative care team.

Prostate cancer – the future

The prospects for significant progress in prostate cancer in the near future are now better than ever. We can hopefully look forward to effective prevention, earlier diagnosis, better staging, and more effective and less toxic therapy. A number of current research endeavours to improve our understanding of the disease may well translate into improved quality of life and improved survival prospects for those affected by prostate cancer.

Chemoprevention

In the future, it may be possible to prevent prostate cancer. Already there is some evidence that both vitamin E and selenium may have a preventative effect (see pages 5 and 6). The benefits of the 5-alpha-reductase inhibitor Avodart (dutasteride) are also currently being assessed in the large REDUCE trial, and several other agents, such as statins which are currently used to lower cholesterol, appear to show promise, but require further research to ensure their safety and effectiveness.

Better diagnosis

Earlier detection, while the disease is still curable, is already a reality as a result of PSA testing. In the future, new tests or variations of existing tests will continue to improve the ability of doctors and surgeons to distinguish early prostate cancer from BPH. Recently, a new test for prostate cancer called the PCA3 (prostate cancer antigen 3) test has been described. It is based on a special genetic analysis of prostate cancer cells present in the urine immediately after a thorough massage of the prostate gland. Preliminary studies suggest that it may be more accurate than the PSA test, but much more research is needed before the true value of this test is known.

www.prostate-research.org.uk

It also seems likely that tests will soon be developed that predict the behaviour of individual prostate cancers more accurately, which will make it easier for patients, their family and their doctors to decide which is the best treatment option.

New treatments

Cryotherapy
Cryotherapy uses freezing to destroy the prostatic tissue. An ultrasound probe in the rectum enables the position of the prostate to be seen on a computer screen. A number of 'cryogenic' probes are then inserted into the prostate, and liquid nitrogen is circulated to reduce the temperature to around –180°C. At this temperature, the tissue surrounding the probes is destroyed. The urethra is protected by circulating warm water through a catheter. Some studies have

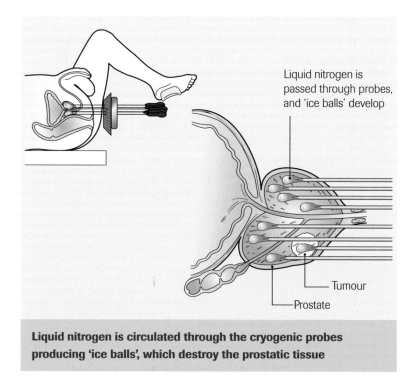

Liquid nitrogen is passed through probes, and 'ice balls' develop

Tumour

Prostate

Liquid nitrogen is circulated through the cryogenic probes producing 'ice balls', which destroy the prostatic tissue

reported survival rates similar to those achieved with radical prostatectomy, but others have described rectal and urethral damage, which can be difficult to repair. No long-term randomized controlled trials to compare cryotherapy with established treatments have yet been carried out. Currently, it is mainly used as a treatment for prostate cancer that has recurred after radiotherapy, since other treatment options in that situation are limited and the technique does offer the potential of cure. Some surgeons are, however, starting to use it as a primary treatment for patients with locally advanced cancers who wish to avoid radiotherapy.

High-intensity focused ultrasound (HIFU)

HIFU is a new technology that allows ultrasound waves to be focused on prostate cancer cells. It involves the insertion of an ultrasound probe into the rectum under anaesthesia and then the destruction of the cancer cells by ultrasound energy; the treatment can take up to 3 hours. It can be used to treat both newly diagnosed cancers and recurrences after radiotherapy. Initial results look encouraging, since the PSA levels seem to decline and side effects are not prominent, although a catheter is required for several days and sometimes longer after treatment because the prostate swells in response to therapy. Damage to the bladder and rectum have been described as a result of HIFU, so you should seek out a team with extensive experience with this technique if you are considering this as an option. Much longer-term follow-up and trials comparing it with surgery and radiotherapy will be required before HIFU can be regarded as a mainstream treatment, but early results are positive.

Drug treatments

As new anti-androgens are developed, it is likely that they will be used at earlier stages of the disease when the cancer cells are more sensitive to the blocking of the action of testosterone.

Research is also being carried out into several drugs that block the pathways of the growth factors that are necessary for the development and progression of prostate cancer. In order

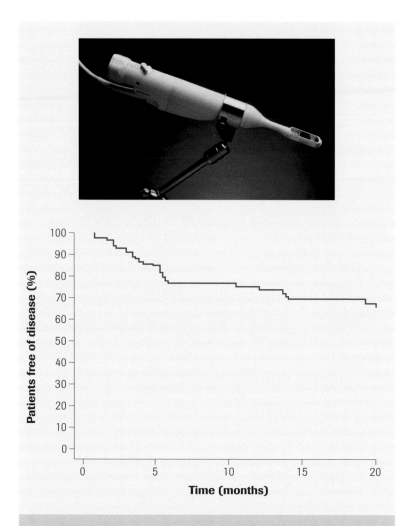

The HIFU probe is inserted into the rectum so that ultrasound waves can be focused on the cancer cells in the prostate. The results of treatment look promising so far in terms of the length of time before the cancer recurs

for a cancer to grow, it requires a new blood supply. Drugs that block the growth of this blood supply have anticancer potential. These so-called angiogenesis inhibitors are currently being tested for activity against prostate cancer. Many of these new approaches offer the possibility of fewer side effects and greater effectiveness.

Immunotherapy

Work on harnessing the immune system to counter prostate cancer may eventually make it possible to vaccinate men at high risk of the disease or induce an immune response against established disease.

Gene therapy

Spectacular advances in molecular biology have made the prospect of gene therapy an imminent reality. In the not too distant future, it may be possible to 'turn off' the oncogenes that induce cancer and 'turn on' the protective tumour suppressor genes. New therapies will also be developed that selectively destroy prostate cancer by activating the in-built cell suicide system known as 'apoptosis'.

BPH – its symptoms, diagnosis and treatment

Nearly half (around 43%) of men over the age of 65 have either urinary symptoms or a reduced urinary flow due to benign prostatic hyperplasia (BPH). BPH is characterized by the benign (non-cancerous) overgrowth of prostate cells, with the effect that the middle portion of the prostate progressively enlarges. The result is that the part of the urethra that is surrounded by the prostate becomes constricted. This reduces the urinary flow and the man finds that his urine stream becomes weaker and it is more difficult to empty his bladder. These symptoms may significantly impair quality of life.

In response to the increasing obstruction, the bladder's walls, which are muscular, thicken and become stronger. Consequently, the pressure inside the bladder needed to produce urinary flow has to increase to overcome the effect of the obstruction; this high pressure causes pouches or 'diverticula' to form. Less commonly, the raised pressure results in what is known as 'back pressure' on the kidneys, causing kidney problems. If BPH is not treated, either chronic urinary retention (characterized by a massively over-distended bladder) or acute urinary retention (the sudden and painful inability to pass any urine) may develop. In either situation, hospital admission, catheterization and eventually prostate surgery are usually required.

Why do some men suffer more than others?

Recent work has clarified the risk factors linked to an increased likelihood of developing complications of BPH. The larger the prostate (as assessed by digital rectal examination), the greater the risk. Similarly, the risk is increased among those men with a PSA level above 1.4 ng/mL. In fact the higher the PSA (provided prostate cancer is not present), the greater the risk of

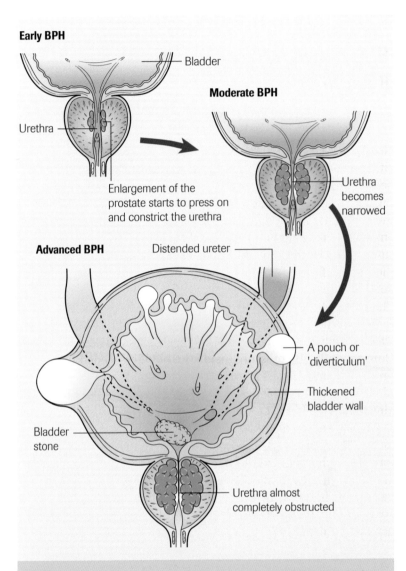

Early BPH

Bladder

Urethra

Enlargement of the
prostate starts to press on
and constrict the urethra

Moderate BPH

Urethra
becomes
narrowed

Advanced BPH

Distended ureter

A pouch or
'diverticulum'

Thickened
bladder wall

Bladder
stone

Urethra almost
completely obstructed

**BPH arises as a consequence of excess non-cancerous growth
of prostate tissue. The urethra running through the prostate
becomes squeezed and the urine flow becomes obstructed.
Because the pressure inside the bladder also builds up, the
bladder walls become thickened and diverticula can form.
Bladder stones can also occur as a result of this condition**

73

Why you may be referred to a specialist

- Your symptoms appeared suddenly or are severe

- You have had repeated urinary infections

- You have passed blood in your urine

- Your PSA level is over 4 ng/mL (2.5 ng/mL in younger men)

- Your GP thinks you may have a bladder stone

- The results from your blood tests suggest you might have kidney damage

retention. Also more likely to develop complications are men whose urine tends to flow slowly and those who have a relatively large amount of urine left in their bladder after attempting to urinate. Although not all men suffer progressive deterioration, in the majority of cases the symptoms gradually become worse over time and eventually complications develop.

How is BPH diagnosed?

The spectrum of symptoms that are associated with BPH are known collectively as lower urinary tract symptoms (LUTS for short), and are outlined in the table below.

The symptoms of BPH overlap with those of other conditions, so your initial examination should be thorough and your doctor will question you about your general health and symptoms. In order to assess your symptoms systematically, you may be asked questions that relate to a scoring system (an example of this system is shown on page 24). Your doctor will also be concerned with how 'bothersome' you find your symptoms. Again, this can be approached in a systematic manner, and your responses can be scored. Enquiries will be made about other conditions, such as diabetes and hypertension, and what medications you are taking.

Lower urinary tract symptoms associated with BPH

- Hesitancy (when the urine flow stops and starts)

- A weak urine stream

- You need to strain to pass urine

- Urination takes a long time

- After urinating, you feel as though there is still some urine 'left behind' in the bladder

- When you get the urge to urinate, you feel you need to do so urgently

- Frequent trips to the toilet

- Getting up in the night to urinate

- When you get the urge to urinate, you leak a little urine

- A sudden or slowly building inability to urinate

Physical examination and digital rectal examination

A digital rectal examination will be performed to give the doctor an idea of the size and consistency of your prostate (see page 22). He will also feel your abdomen to check whether your bladder is distended so that it can be felt (if it can, this is a sign that you may be retaining urine). Your doctor may also make an assessment of your nervous system, such as testing the muscle tone and sensation in the area around and between the scrotum and anus, as some disorders of the nervous system, such as Parkinson's disease, can give rise to urinary symptoms similar to those of BPH. Since high blood pressure (hypertension) is common, blood pressure may also be measured as part of a general health check.

Urine test

As a urinary tract infection can cause symptoms such as an increased need to urinate, a urine sample will be checked for signs of bacterial infection or blood. The urine may also be tested routinely for the presence of sugar, which is a sign of diabetes.

Blood tests

A very small proportion of men have kidney problems as a consequence of their BPH. By assessing the amount of a substance called creatinine in the blood, your doctor will be able to check whether your kidneys are affected. Your blood sugar level may also be tested to check that you do not have diabetes, as this can be a cause of frequent urination.

The amount of PSA may also be measured. You might already have read about this in the sections on prostate cancer. PSA is a marker that indicates damage to the prostate, often arising as a result of prostate cancer, but sometimes as a result of BPH. In fact, the larger your prostate, the higher your PSA tends to be. If your PSA level is raised, it may be recommended that you have a prostate biopsy so that prostate cancer can be excluded (see pages 26 and 27). As already mentioned, your PSA level also gives a rough indication of your prostate size, and this can influence the risk of you developing urinary retention and provide information about the likely success of various medical treatment options.

Urine flow tests (or uroflowmetry)

By measuring the speed of your urine output over time, your urologist can get some useful information about your urine flow. For this test you will have to urinate into the bowl of a specialized piece of medical equipment known as a flow meter.

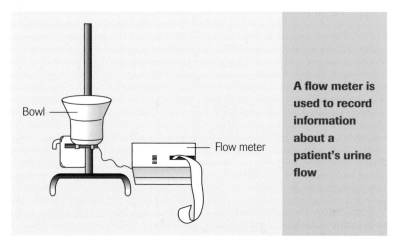

Bowl

Flow meter

A flow meter is used to record information about a patient's urine flow

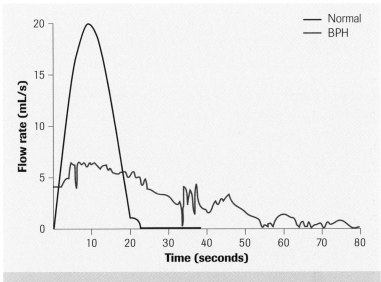

The urine flow rate in men with BPH is slower than normal and lasts longer

Ultrasound to measure urine left in the bladder

Ultrasound can give your doctor an idea of how severe the obstruction is and how well you might respond to certain types of treatment. The procedure is very similar to that used for pregnant women. High-frequency sound waves are emitted from a probe that is passed over your abdomen, and the echoes build up a picture that can be seen on a computer monitor.

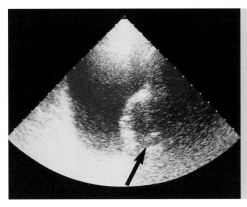

An ultrasound image of the bladder showing that a large volume of urine remains in the bladder after the patient has urinated. In this example, the prostate can be seen bulging into the base of the bladder (arrowed)

77

Less common tests

Depending on the results of the tests already described, your urologist may want to perform some further tests.

Urodynamic measurements are made using a small catheter that is inserted up through the urethra, via your penis, into the bladder. By measuring the pressure within your bladder, your urologist can deduce whether your symptoms are due to obstruction from BPH or are the result of the bladder itself not working properly. This test is uncomfortable rather than painful, and takes around 20 minutes.

Transrectal ultrasonography (TRUS) is used to visualize the prostate, measure its proportions and help guide a biopsy needle when there is a possibility of prostate cancer. The procedure is described fully on pages 25 and 26.

Treatment

BPH is most commonly treated with drugs or surgery. Some men with very mild symptoms opt for active surveillance (or watchful waiting), which involves monitoring their condition so that any worsening can be quickly spotted and treated. There are also several 'minimally invasive' alternatives, though many of these are relatively new and long-term experience with them is limited.

Drug treatment

Drug treatment may be recommended if your symptoms are moderate, though it may also be beneficial for patients with severe symptoms. Certain complications of BPH, such as kidney problems, urinary retention or bladder stones, make surgery a more appropriate option.

There are two main classes of drug that are prescribed for BPH:

- alpha-blockers
- 5-alpha-reductase inhibitors.

Alpha-blockers work by helping to relax the muscles at the neck of the bladder and in the prostate. By reducing the

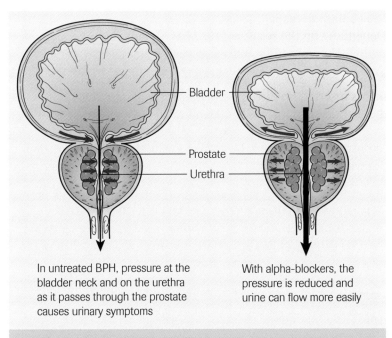

In untreated BPH, pressure at the bladder neck and on the urethra as it passes through the prostate causes urinary symptoms

With alpha-blockers, the pressure is reduced and urine can flow more easily

Alpha-blockers relax the muscles at the neck of the bladder and in the prostate, so reducing the pressure on the urethra

pressure on the urethra, they help to overcome the obstruction and so increase the flow of urine. Results available from studies to date indicate that up to 60% of men find that their symptoms improve significantly within the first 2–3 weeks of treatment with an alpha-blocker.

This type of drug does not cure BPH, but simply helps to alleviate some of the symptoms. You may still develop complications at a later date and you may still need surgery eventually.

The most commonly occurring side effects are tiredness, dizziness and headache, which affect around one in ten men. The dosage of earlier alpha-blockers had to be increased gradually to reduce the likelihood of side effects, but this is not necessary with more recently developed drugs, such as Flomaxtra (tamsulosin) or Xatral (alfuzosin), which seem to have fewer side effects.

5-alpha-reductase inhibitors work by blocking the conversion of testosterone to another substance, DHT (dihydrotestosterone), that is known to have a key role in prostate growth. To date, most information is available on the 5-alpha-reductase inhibitor Proscar (finasteride); a newer agent, Avodart (dutasteride) is also now available. Unlike alpha-blockers, Proscar and Avodart do appear to be able to reverse the condition to some extent, particularly if the prostate is significantly enlarged, so its use may reduce the likelihood that you will develop acute urinary retention and eventually require surgery. These drugs also seem to work better in patients with larger glands, but it can take 6 months or so for them to be effective. Importantly, they do reduce the PSA value by around 50% so this should be taken into account when monitoring for prostate cancer; one way to do this is to double the PSA value obtained when a patient is taking either Avodart or Proscar.

The main side effects of these agents are a reduced sex drive and difficulty in maintaining/achieving an erection; these appear to affect around 3–5 men in every 100. There is also a small chance of about 1% or less that you might experience tenderness and swelling around the nipples. These symptoms usually disappear if treatment is stopped. Be aware that crushed or broken Proscar or Avodart tablets should not be handled by a woman who is pregnant or who is planning a pregnancy, as there is a risk that they could cause problems to a developing baby.

Combination therapy with an alpha-blocker or a 5-alpha-reductase inhibitor has been shown (in the Medical Treatment of Prostate Symptoms study) to be more effective than either agent used alone in preventing the worsening of the symptoms of BPH or the development of complications, such as acute retention or the need for surgery. However, the increased cost and additional side effects have to be weighed against these benefits. Patients most likely to respond to combination therapy are those with both a large prostate and severe symptoms.

Other medical strategies for symptom relief in BPH include anticholinergic agents like Detrusitol XL (tolterodine) and

Vesicare (solifenacin) to control urinary urgency and frequency. However, these agents carry a small risk of precipitating acute retention of urine in men with severe obstruction and may also result in a dry mouth. Very recently, Botox (Botulinum toxin) has been used in a small number of men with BPH in the form of an injection into the prostate under ultrasound control. Preliminary results look encouraging, but the results of larger, longer studies are needed before it can be regarded as standard therapy.

In patients who are particularly troubled by the need to pass urine during the night (nocturia), vasopressin analogues such as Desmospray or Desmotabs (desmopressin) last thing at night, used in addition to fluid restriction in the evenings, can be quite effective. These drugs work by reducing the amount of urine produced by the kidneys for 6–8 hours.

Surgery

There are a number of surgical options for BPH:

- transurethral resection of the prostate (TURP)
- transurethral incision of the prostate (TUIP)
- open prostatectomy
- laser prostatectomy.

TURP is the most usual operation for men who have not responded to medical therapy or who have developed complications such as complete retention of urine, and is usually carried out under a general anaesthetic. It involves passing an instrument up through the penis, and then using it to cut the middle out of the enlarged prostate, piecemeal (see diagram overleaf). A catheter will be passed through the urethra into the bladder at the end of the operation to drain off the urine. This will be left in place for a couple of days. A normal hospital stay following TURP is 3 or 4 days, but you should try to rest as much as possible for a few weeks afterwards to minimize the risk of secondary complications such as bleeding that may occur 10–12 days after the original operation.

After the operation, you may find that you experience an urgent need to urinate and/or a burning sensation when you

81

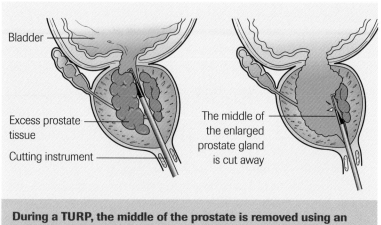

Bladder

Excess prostate
tissue

The middle of
the enlarged
prostate gland
is cut away

Cutting instrument

During a TURP, the middle of the prostate is removed using an instrument passed through the urethra

pass urine. This should disappear within a few weeks. You may also notice some blood in your urine. This is normal, but if it is particularly heavy or persists for more than a few weeks, or if you notice some blood clots, drink extra fluids and contact your doctor.

The most common side effect is a phenomenon known as retrograde ejaculation – where semen passes into the bladder during orgasm, rather than out through the penis. You then pass the semen mixed with urine the next time you urinate. This is not harmful and, providing that they know about this potential side effect before undergoing the surgery, most men do not find it bothersome. However, retrograde ejaculation may reduce your fertility, though it does not make you reliably sterile.

A few men complain of an inability to achieve or maintain an erection after the operation, though this does not seem to be a problem specifically caused by this surgical procedure. In a study that compared men with BPH who had undergone a TURP with men with BPH who had not had surgery, the proportions of men who reported erectile problems were similar. Some were even improved by surgery.

Some men notice some incontinence after a TURP – if you find that you are leaking urine slightly, talk to your doctor. This

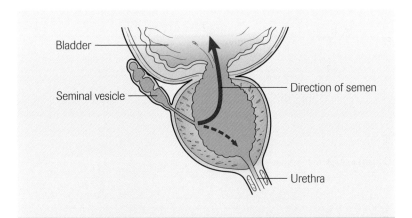

Bladder

Seminal vesicle

Direction of semen

Urethra

Retrograde ejaculation is a common side effect of a TURP. Semen passes into the bladder rather than out through the urethra and penis at orgasm

problem nearly always resolves completely with time, but if it persists further investigation may be warranted.

An operation under general anaesthetic always carries some small risks, as occasionally an individual reacts badly to anaesthesia. There is also a small chance of significant blood loss and the subsequent need for a transfusion. In the postoperative period, there may be problems with catheter blockage or bleeding after the catheter has been removed. These problems are relatively unusual with a TURP, however, and the outcome is usually good.

When a TURP is performed the prostate tissue removed is sent to the pathology laboratory for analysis. In most cases the results come back confirming benign prostatic hyperplasia (BPH); however, in around one case in ten, a small amount of prostate cancer is identified. Small areas of prostate cancer may not require active treatment, but careful follow-up is indicated and biopsy of the remaining prostate tissue should be considered, as it may harbour some residual cancer tissue.

TUIP is appropriate for the man who is experiencing obstruction problems but who has a relatively small prostate. It is quite quick to perform, taking only around 20 minutes, but

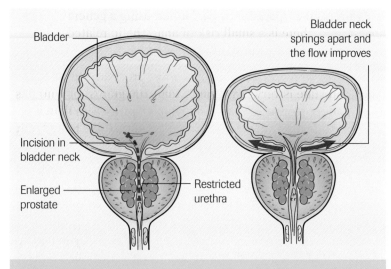

Bladder

Bladder neck
springs apart and
the flow improves

Incision in
bladder neck

Enlarged
prostate

Restricted
urethra

In TUIP, several small cuts are made in the bladder neck and prostate. This relieves the pressure on the urethra and urine can flow more easily

you will still be given a general or spinal anaesthetic. As with a TURP, an instrument will be passed up through the penis, but with a TUIP, rather than removing a portion of the prostate, one or two small cuts are made in the neck of the bladder and in the prostate. These have the effect of reducing the obstruction and allowing the bladder neck to spring apart. As with a TURP, you will be catheterized at the end of the operation to allow urine to drain away freely. The catheter will be removed after around 24–48 hours, and you will be able to leave hospital after a couple of days. For the next week or so, you should take things easy.

The chance that you will experience a side effect following a TUIP is lower than following a TURP. Retrograde ejaculation (see pages 82 and 83), for example, affects a much lower proportion of men after the operation (one in ten compared with eight in ten).

There is a risk that symptoms will return after the operation (see table on page 86); if this happens, then it is likely that you will need a TURP.

Again, as the operation is performed using a general anaesthetic, there is a small risk of anaesthetic-related complications and postoperative bleeding.

Open prostatectomy is only really appropriate for the man whose prostate is very large (more than 100 grams) or who has large bladder stones. It is a more complex procedure than a TURP, and complications afterwards are somewhat more likely.

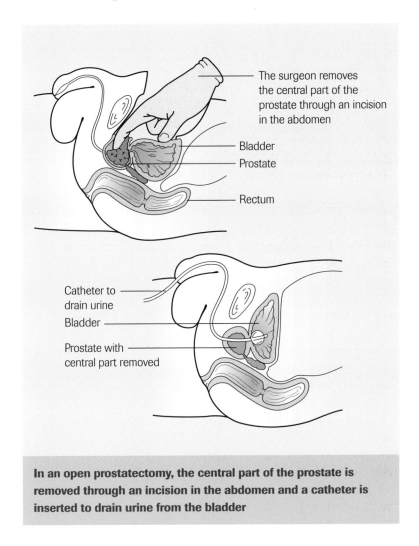

The surgeon removes the central part of the prostate through an incision in the abdomen

Bladder
Prostate
Rectum

Catheter to drain urine
Bladder
Prostate with central part removed

In an open prostatectomy, the central part of the prostate is removed through an incision in the abdomen and a catheter is inserted to drain urine from the bladder

The surgeon gains access to the prostate through a horizontal incision made in the lower abdomen. Through a cut made either in the prostate or bladder, the surgeon is then able to remove the central part of the prostate. A catheter will be inserted into your bladder during the operation so that urine can drain away, and this will be left in place for 3 or 4 days. Because this is relatively major surgery, you will usually need to stay in hospital for about a week. Even when you go home, you are advised to rest for up to 6 weeks, and you should avoid lifting anything heavy for several months. The operation will leave a scar.

An open prostatectomy can also result in retrograde ejaculation (see pages 82 and 83), with about seven in ten men being affected; some men also find it difficult to achieve/maintain an erection (around two men in ten). The risks associated with surgery of this type are discussed in the TURP section.

The long-term picture following surgery
Useful information comparing the outcomes following each surgical procedure is presented in the table.

Outcome after the three main surgical options for treatment of BPH			
	TURP	**TUIP**	**Open prostatectomy**
Likelihood that symptoms will improve	90%	80%	98%
Usual reduction in symptom score (see page 23)	85%	73%	79%
Likelihood that you will need further surgery within 8 years	16–20%	Over 20%	10%

Active surveillance
Active surveillance (watchful waiting) may be recommended if your symptoms are mild or if you are not too troubled by them.

Your doctor will advise you about small changes that you can make to your lifestyle that might help; for example, try not to drink large volumes of fluid in the evenings. Tea, coffee and alcohol can worsen symptoms. At regular intervals (usually yearly) you will have a check up that will include the examination and tests described on pages 21 and 22.

Newer minimally invasive treatments

As has already been said, minimally invasive treatments are relatively new. While greeted with enthusiasm by some urologists – and many patients – it has to be said that, currently, minimally invasive techniques do not always work as well (or as definitively) as the more traditional treatments. Two that particularly deserve a mention are transurethral microwave thermotherapy and laser therapy.

Transurethral microwave thermotherapy involves using microwave energy to generate heat, which then destroys some of the prostate tissue. Under local anaesthetic, the microwave device is inserted up through the urethra inside a rigid catheter; the temperature of surrounding tissues is monitored using a probe inserted in the rectum. A catheter may be necessary for a few days because of the swelling of the gland in response to the heat.

Laser therapy is carried out under general anaesthetic. A laser probe is inserted up through the penis, and the laser energy it generates destroys some of the prostate tissue. Green-light laser vaporizes the prostate so that no tissue is available for examination under the microscope. A new holmium laser technique – so-called holmium laser enucleation of the prostate or HoLEP – allows the prostate to be cut away, and the pieces are then broken down into a paste and removed from the bladder by suction. Bleeding is minimal after laser therapy, but catheterization is usually necessary for a short time afterwards. For a while, a burning sensation may be experienced on passing urine, which may be prolonged and quite troublesome. If this persists, a urine specimen should be sent to the laboratory for culture to rule out a urinary tract infection. The laser techniques are especially suitable for patients taking anticoagulants because they cause virtually no bleeding and are becoming more popular as more and more specialized laser machines become available. What is not quite clear yet is how durable this treatment is in the longer term.

Plant extracts (phytotherapy)

There is an increasing range of plant extracts available that supposedly alleviate BPH and many claims have been made for their effectiveness. However, scientific data from properly conducted, long-term studies to support their safety and usefulness are limited. A recent report on saw palmetto suggested that it was no more effective than inactive placebo; however, some patients swear by it. Nevertheless, phytotherapy almost certainly does no harm, it is relatively cheap and most urologists do not actively discourage its use.

Prevention

Although we have still to identify the fundamental steps in the development of BPH, we know that testosterone is certainly involved in some way and it is likely that the female hormone oestrogen also has a role. Epidemiological data suggest that men in the Far East are protected, to some extent, against the risks of BPH by minute amounts of oestrogen-like substances in the food that they eat (for example, soya contains the phytoestrogen genistein). This raises the question as to whether dietary supplements taken regularly by men in Europe, the USA and elsewhere could protect against the risk of this disease. Long-term studies involving many men are needed to confirm this.

Case study

Edward, a 58-year-old designer, noticed a gradual diminution of his urinary stream and a feeling of incomplete bladder emptying. He was also getting up two or three times per night to pass urine. He consulted his GP who examined him and found a smoothly enlarged prostate, and checked his PSA and found it normal at 2.6 ng/mL. He was started on an alpha-blocker known as Flowmaxtra (tamsulosin), 0.4 mg/day, and the 5-alpha-reductase inhibitor Avodart (dutasteride), 0.5 mg/day, as combination therapy, and some improvement was noted.

After 8 months, however, he returned to his doctor and requested a referral to a urologist as he was still getting up at night and consequently feeling tired during the day. He was seen promptly, and a flow test and bladder ultrasound confirmed that he was still obstructed with a slow flow and incomplete bladder empting. A TURP was advised and this was accomplished uneventfully. Pathological examination of the prostate tissue removed confirmed BPH. Subsequently Edward passed urine less frequently with a much improved flow. Although he did develop retrograde ejaculation, this has not proved bothersome to him and he is happy with the outcome of treatment.

Prostatitis – the painful prostate

Prostatitis literally means 'inflammation of the prostate'. In fact, by no means every patient suffering from prostatitis actually has an inflamed prostate, so the name is rather misleading. In the UK, the condition accounts for almost one-quarter of all consultations with a urologist.

Patients with prostatitis often suffer pain and discomfort in the area around and between the anus and scrotum, and just above the pubic bone. Men with the condition may have to urinate frequently and this can be very inconvenient. There may also be a burning sensation at the time of urination and/or some discomfort during or after ejaculation (see the table below for a more complete list of symptoms). Although prostatitis is often considered to be the result of a bacterial infection in the prostate, inflammation, when present, more

Symptoms of prostatitis

- Chills and fever
- Pain in:
    - lower back (may be particularly painful after sex)
    - between the scrotum and rectum
    - penis
    - prostate (felt as lower abdominal pain and pain in the area between the scrotum and anus)
    - testicles
    - rectum
    - inner thighs
- Pain/difficulty in passing urine
- A need for frequent urination

Classification of prostatitis (National Institutes of Health, USA)

Category I – acute bacterial prostatitis

Acute bacterial prostatitis is usually caused by a bacterial urinary tract infection and is the least common, but most severe, form of prostatitis. Sufferers can feel generally unwell.

Category II – chronic bacterial prostatitis

Chronic bacterial prostatitis is a chronic or recurrent infection of the prostate that may be present for several years before any symptoms develop. The symptoms may be less aggressive, but are recurring.

Category III – chronic (abacterial) prostatitis

- IIIA: inflammatory (chronic pelvic pain syndrome)

- IIIb: non-inflammatory (prostatodynia)

Chronic (abacterial) prostatitis is the most common form of prostatitis and is a recurring (relapsing) condition. It is difficult to pinpoint a specific cause for this condition, but it is thought that an abnormal immune system reaction or a chemical reaction to urine flowing backwards into the prostatic ducts could play a major role. Earlier suggestions that some sexually transmitted conditions, such as *Chlamydia* or *Mycoplasma*, might be responsible have been disproved.

Category IV – asymptomatic inflammatory prostatitis

Some men feel discomfort that appears to come from their prostate or the surrounding area without any infection being present. Although there are many theories as to its cause, more research is required, as the inflammation could possibly lead to more serious problems, such as prostate cancer.

commonly occurs spontaneously. Some studies suggest that in the absence of infection, inflammation may result from urine being forced backwards up the prostatic ducts at the time of urination. Recently, the question has been raised as to whether, in the long run, inflammation can lead on eventually to prostate cancer. This is possibly because the inflammatory

91

cells that infiltrate the prostate release chemicals that cause oxidative stress and thereby damage DNA in prostate cells.

Even when infection is the source of inflammation, it may be difficult to eradicate because the bacteria responsible tend to be inaccessible to antibiotics. This is because they usually lurk deep inside the prostate (for example, the bacteria may be inside the tiny stones that form in the prostatic ducts).

Risk factors

Men who have an increased risk of prostatitis include those who have a previous history of the problem or long-term catheterization and those who have urinary tract infections that remain untreated. Some unconventional forms of sex may also spark off a bout of prostatic infection.

Prostatitis most commonly affects men in the age range 30–50 years, but a man of any age can be affected. In fact, most men afflicted have no identifiable risk factors.

Tests

Because prostatitis is often the result of a bacterial infection, your doctor will usually want to check a sample of your urine and prostatic secretions for bacteria (the sample will be sent to the laboratory for analysis, so you will not get the results straight away).

Obtaining a sample of prostatic secretions

You will be asked to pass urine and provide a sample. Your prostate will then be massaged so that secretions are released, which will be collected from the urethra into a sterile pot. Although this process is unquestionably a little uncomfortable, it is not actually painful. Finally, a second urine sample will be collected. If there is a bacterial infection, bacteria can be grown up in the laboratory from cultures of the prostatic secretions and the second urine sample. This method also allows the specific type of bacteria responsible to be identified, and an appropriate antibiotic to be prescribed.

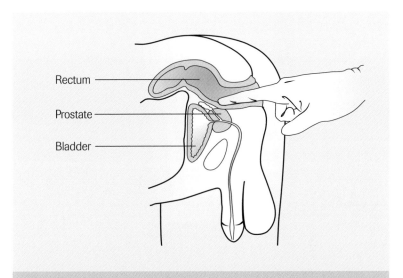

Rectum

Prostate

Bladder

Prostatic massage. The patient is asked to pass urine and a specimen is taken for culture. The prostate is then massaged and any secretions produced are also sent to the laboratory. Finally, a further urine sample is collected that also contains fluid expressed from the prostate

Other tests

Depending on your symptoms, your doctor may also check that you do not have BPH or prostate cancer – the tests that may be performed are discussed on pages 21–22 and 75–78. Remember that prostatitis, particularly when the inflammation is severe, may sometimes cause a temporary increase in blood PSA level (see page 12). Prostatitis can also cause blood flow in the prostate to become increased, and this can show up when a transrectal ultrasound study of the prostate is performed using what is known as a colour Doppler probe.

If a prostatic abscess is suspected, a CT scan may be arranged to confirm or exclude a collection of pus in the prostate.

Treatment

If a bacterial infection is the cause of your symptoms, you will be prescribed a course of appropriate antibiotics. You may need

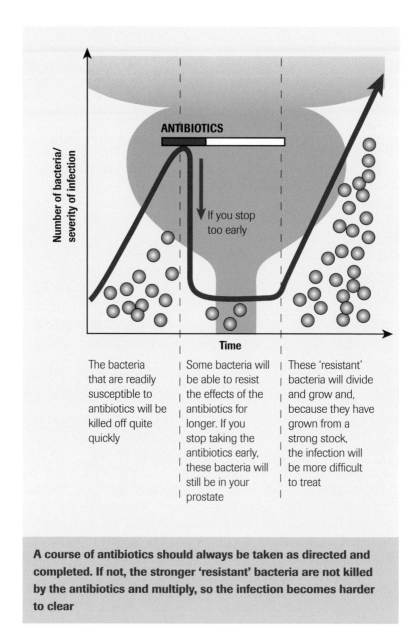

A course of antibiotics should always be taken as directed and completed. If not, the stronger 'resistant' bacteria are not killed by the antibiotics and multiply, so the infection becomes harder to clear

to take these for a relatively long period, often 4–6 weeks, and it is very important that you complete the course (the diagram above explains why this is so). You may also be prescribed an anti-inflammatory drug, such as Voltarol (diclofenac), to reduce the inflammation in the prostate. Remember that these drugs can cause indigestion and bleeding from the stomach, so you should always take them with a meal.

If bacteria are not demonstrably present, you may be given an anti-inflammatory drug in isolation. You may also find that prostatic massage performed by your doctor helps (see page 93). Antibiotics can also be helpful in these circumstances, perhaps because the cultures do not tell the whole story, as the bacteria may be lurking within prostate stones or elsewhere deep within the gland.

Prostatitis, though troublesome, is not a life-threatening condition and is not proven to be a precursor to either BPH or prostate cancer. You may find that, over the years, the prostatitis returns from time to time (particularly if the condition has a non-bacterial cause), but your doctor should be able to help alleviate the symptoms quite effectively, so do not suffer in silence. The condition can be frustrating for patient and doctor alike; however, there is some evidence that lifestyle improvements, particularly dietary modification and fitness enhancement, can increase natural immunity and reduce the risk of relapse.

Prostatic abscess

Occasionally prostatitis with a bacterial cause can lead to the formation of an abscess within the prostate itself. If this is the case, your doctor may need to take a sample of fluid from the abscess and will do so using ultrasound for guidance (see page 27). The sample can then be checked to see what type of bacteria has caused the infection, so that appropriate antibiotics can be given.

Abscesses sometimes have to be drained, which involves passing an instrument up through the penis under anaesthetic, making a small cut through to the abscess and then 'nicking' the abscess to allow pus to drain out. A course of antibiotics and a period of catheterization are also often necessary as passing urine can difficult or impossible, because of the associated swelling.

Preventing prostatitis

Prostatitis is the affliction of the prostate about which we know least. So, not surprisingly, we currently have little idea how to prevent the problem. The best advice at present is to avoid the risk factors for prostatitis where possible (for example, if you have symptoms of a urinary tract infection, such as a burning sensation when urinating, or cloudy, smelly urine, visit your doctor and complete any prescribed courses of antibiotics). Also, maintain a healthy lifestyle, eat a diet low in saturated fats, take plenty of exercise and always be vigilant about avoiding a risk of infection, especially during any unorthodox sexual encounter.

Pain but no inflammation: prostatodynia

Some men feel pain that appears to come from their prostate or the surrounding area, but investigation does not appear to reveal any inflammation or infection. What causes this condition, which is referred to as prostatodynia or pelvic pain syndrome, is not known, though it may result from spasm of the pelvic muscles brought on by stress and anxiety. Depending on your symptoms, you may be given alpha-blockers (see pages 78 and 79), which may have to be taken for some time, or the muscle relaxant diazepam. Much more research is needed into this disorder to identify the underlying cause of the problem, to improve the cure rate and enhance the quality of life of those affected.

Case study

Matthew, a bond dealer aged 34, presented to his urologist with a long history of intermittent pelvic and perineal pain, together with bouts of frequency of urination. Several courses of antibiotics including ampicillin and oxytetracycline had only resulted in temporary improvement. He was eventually referred to a urologist who found a tender prostate on examination and sent some prostatic secretions off for culture. These came back showing inflammatory cells, but no bacterial growth. A 6-week course of Ciproxin (ciprofloxacin) and Brufen (ibuprofen) was prescribed and lifestyle modification advised. The medications, in addition to the running, swimming, cycling and the improved diet, resulted in a marked improvement. Matthew has been warned, however, that relapse is possible and is therefore resolved to maintain the changes in his lifestyle.

Treatment of your prostate problem: some practical advice

Emergency? When to call your doctor

- If you find that you suddenly cannot pass urine yet your bladder is full.
- If you have had a biopsy or operation, and develop symptoms of infection:
  - high temperature
  - pain on urination
  - cloudy, smelly urine
  - swollen or painful testicles.
- If you have a catheter in place and notice that urine does not drain into the collecting bag for several hours.
- If you suddenly start to pass blood in your urine. Drink extra fluids and call your doctor. If clots start to form, there is a risk that you will be unable to pass urine, in which case you will need to go to hospital urgently to have a catheter inserted via the penis to drain urine from your bladder.

Having an operation

Consent. By signing a consent form, you are formally agreeing to undergo the treatment specified on the form. So do not sign it lightly.

- Be sure that you know what the operation involves, what the side effects and risks are, and what effect the operation will have on the course of your illness.
- Be aware that you may need to undergo an investigation of your prostate and bladder carried out under general anaesthetic.
- Ask who will be performing the surgery and who will be around afterwards.

If you are not completely satisfied, do not sign the form.

Talking to the anaesthetist. Before your operation, you will meet your anaesthetist. He is a fully trained doctor who has specialized in the administration of anaesthetics. You might be asked some of the following questions about your medical history.

- Have you had surgery before? If so, were there any problems or complications?
- Has any member of your family had a problem following an operation?
- Are you taking any medicines that have been prescribed to you or that you bought from a chemist, such as aspirin or Plavix (clopidogrel) or warfarin?
- Do you or any member of your family have any allergies (for example, to plasters or antibiotics)?
- Do you have any back, chest or heart problems?
- Do you smoke?

The anaesthetist will also ask about your teeth. This may seem a strange line of questioning, but he needs to know whether there is anything in your mouth, such as a cap or a crown, that might come loose during the operation.

Do not be afraid to ask him about any questions or concerns that you may have.

Physical appearance

Some men feel that their penis appears shorter in length after radical prostatectomy, though not in circumference. However, it is somewhat relative. If there is a noticeable difference, it is very slight. It happens because the newly sutured urethra has been necessarily shortened and therefore had the effect of 'pulling back' the penis into the body just a little.

After a few months, the urethra will stretch to accommodate most of the change. On erection, the difference is usually of little or no consequence.

Eating and drinking

If you have had an operation, whether open, transurethral or laparoscopic, you will probably feel tired and sore. It is a good idea to eat foods that will help you to avoid constipation, so that you do not have to strain to empty your bowels. Eat sensibly, including plenty of fresh and dried fruit (for example, prunes), fresh vegetables, wholemeal bread and high-fibre breakfast cereals, such as All-Bran, in your diet. Laxatives such as Milpar may also be helpful.

Also keep your fluid intake up – try to drink 2 litres (more than 3 pints) a day if possible. This may take a bit of readjustment as you might have reduced the amount you drank before your operation in an effort to keep the number of trips to the toilet down. Water or flavoured squash drinks are fine, but try not to overdo your intake of tea, coffee or cola. It is also worth trying cranberry juice, as this probably reduces the likelihood of urinary tract infections (it is thought to work by making the environment of the bladder and urethra unfavourable to bacteria).

Looking after a catheter

If you have a catheter inserted during surgery (for example following a radical prostatectomy or HIFU) and have to keep it for a few days after you have been sent home, it is important to keep it clean. The hospital staff will probably have shown you how to do this, so this short section should act as a reminder.

The catheter itself. The catheter must be kept clean. If possible, always wash your hands before touching it or any part of the system. Twice a day, wash the area of skin where the catheter enters your body with soap and water, and then dry it thoroughly. Do not use anything else, such as talc, around this area.

The catheter is held in place by a Velcro strap, which fits around the catheter and your leg, and prevents it from being pulled.

The leg bag is securely attached to your leg by a leg-bag support, which is rather like a sock. The leg bag will fill with urine during the day and you will feel it getting heavier as it fills. Do not let it become too full – open the tap over the toilet and drain the urine from the bag at regular intervals. Always wash your hands before and after doing this.

The night bag should be attached to the bottom of the leg bag, and the tap should be opened to allow urine to drain into the night bag, which should be attached to a stand (you will have to be shown how to do this). In the morning, do not forget to close the tap before removing the night bag. After disposing of the urine, rinse the night bag with warm water so that it is ready to be used again the next night.

Changing bags. Unless there is a problem, only change your catheter bag once a week. To dispose of a bag, empty it, rinse it out and put it in a sealed plastic bag with your household waste.

Leakage can occur if the bladder muscle goes into spasm. If you leak a little urine outside of the catheter, check that the connection between the catheter and the leg bag is still good and that urine is still being collected in the leg bag. If it is, then carry on as normal, but let your doctor or nurse know what has happened. If the bladder spasms are very troublesome then removing some of the fluid from the catheter balloon can be very helpful. You will usually need to see your doctor or nurse to sort this out. Alternatively, your doctor may prescribe a drug to reduce bladder contractions, such as Detrusitol XL (tolterodine) or Vesicare (solifenacin).

If urine is not collecting in the bag, check that:
- the bag is below the level of your bladder (if, for example, you are using the night bag on the stand)
- there are no twists or kinks in the catheter.

Also ask yourself whether you have been drinking sufficient fluids or whether you are constipated, as this can be a sign that you are dehydrated. If 1–2 hours pass without any urine draining into the bag, contact your doctor or nurse immediately – the catheter may have become blocked, in which case it will have to be flushed or changed.

Blood in the urine. Blood is commonly seen in the urine after radical prostatectomy. As you become more mobile, the catheter can irritate the bladder and lead to blood in the urine. You may also see blood in the urine when you open your bowels. Do not worry about it unless you can see large clots or pieces of tissue passing down the catheter. These can cause a blockage and you should contact your doctor or nurse for advice.

Infections. You should contact your doctor if you have any of the following symptoms, as they may be due to infection:

- cloudy urine
- a burning sensation (cystitis)
- strong-smelling urine
- a high temperature
- shaking attacks.

Regaining continence

You will probably need to wear a small incontinence pad for a few weeks after a radical prostatectomy. These will be supplied by the team looking after you, and further supplies are available from your GP or can be bought from chemists. After this, if you have had an open or laparoscopic radical prostatectomy, you may find that pelvic floor exercises will help you to regain your continence control.

First you need to become aware of your pelvic floor muscles. Do this in two stages. While passing urine, contract the muscles up and inwards to stop the flow. Then let go. It does not matter if the flow does not stop altogether. The important thing is recognizing the muscles you are using. Once you have done this, there is no need to keep stopping and starting the urine flow. Secondly, tighten the rest of your pelvic floor muscles by pulling up the muscles around your rectum as if to control an attack of diarrhoea.

You should use all of these muscles at the same time when performing pelvic floor exercises. Draw them up and hold them for a count of five, and repeat until you have done five contractions. Try to do this exercise once each hour every day. Do 20 short, sharp contractions every day as well. Try to keep your stomach, thigh and buttock muscles relaxed so that you use only your pelvic floor muscles.

You will probably need to do the regular exercises for several weeks before you notice any improvement. To help you remember to do your exercises, try to schedule each set of contractions to accompany a certain daily task to build them into your routine.

After starting the exercise programme, you may notice a mild aching sensation as the muscles get tired. The ache should disappear within a few days, but you can take a rest from the exercises for a day or two if you wish. However, if you are at all concerned, you should consult your doctor.

Self-catheterization

Occasionally (in up to 8% of cases), narrowing of the bladder neck occurs after radical prostatectomy. This can cause a reduction in the urinary flow and occasionally even complete retention of urine. This problem is simply treated by gently dilating the bladder neck under light sedation, which is sometimes followed by a period of self-catheterization for a few weeks (this involves passing a small slippery tube through the narrowed area on a daily or less frequent basis). These simple measures nearly always resolve the problem, although they sometimes need to be repeated.

Radiotherapy for prostate cancer

Many men opt for radiotherapy for the treatment of their prostate cancer. In general, either external beam radiotherapy or brachytherapy are well tolerated (see page 39). However, the bowel disturbance that accompanies external beam radiotherapy, particularly towards the end of the treatment, can be troublesome. A low-residue diet can help, as can the use of medicines such as codeine phosphate, immodium or lomotil. Rectal bleeding can also occur following treatment and sometimes needs to be treated with Predsol steroid enemas or even laser therapy.

Brachytherapy seldom causes rectal problems but may result in difficulty in passing urine as a result of the swelling of the prostate that follows the insertion of the radioactive seeds. These usually settle eventually, but may persist for some months. Most patients undergoing brachytherapy are prescribed an alpha-blocker, such as Flomaxtra (tamsulosin) or Xatral (alfuzosin), for some time after the implants have been inserted. Occasionally the difficulty in passing urine can be so severe that a catheter is required. In this situation you should consult your doctor urgently.

Sexual problems after treatment

Some treatments for prostate cancer and BPH can leave you with reduced or absent erections (often called erectile dysfunction), although orgasm is usually unaffected. Several drugs to help overcome this problem are now available. The best known is Viagra (sildenafil), but newer drugs, such as Cialis (tadalafil) and Levitra (vardenafil), can also be helpful. Some surgeons are suggesting that they be tried soon after the operation, but they may not work fully until about 6–9 months later. These drugs are, however, not suitable for everyone; for example, if you have angina or had a recent heart attack. In such cases, a number of other options such as silicone implants, inflatable penile prostheses, penile injections of prostaglandin and vacuum pumps can be considered.

Talk to your doctor if you experience loss of erections after treatment. He will be able to advise you about the appropriate options, and give you further information about the pros and cons; do not buy Viagra on the black market – always go through your doctor.

Other considerations

A question that is sometimes posed is: how will my partner be affected? Nobody can 'catch' prostate cancer from you, but your partner will certainly be affected if impotence is the result. Frank discussion is vital before and after the operation, particularly if you go for a radical prostatectomy, and your partner must understand the implications as well as you. Emotional support for a partner and family is just as important as for the sufferer himself, and this is something to which the Prostate Research Campaign UK is firmly committed. In this situation good information is vital, so make sure your partner is as well informed as you are about all facets of prostate treatment.

Some patients ask: should I tell my family and friends I have, or have had, a prostate problem? It is up to you, of course, but why should there be a need for secrecy and shame? In fact, many men feel much better about the problem once they have shared it with their partner and/or close friend. Remember that if you have or have had prostate cancer your first-degree relatives have roughly twice the risk of developing the disease themselves and should therefore be put on their guard. It could also be argued that spreading the word about prostate disease can only help to raise the awareness that is required to help prevent prostate problems ruining people's lives by encouraging them to see a doctor earlier.

Medications commonly used to treat prostate disorders

Alpha-blockers

Alpha-blockers are used in BPH to help relax the muscles in the bladder and the prostate, which in turn helps to reduce the pressure on the urethra. Side effects include headaches, dizziness and nasal stuffiness.

Alpha-blocker	Brand name	Recommended dose
Indoramin	Doralese	20 mg twice daily
Prazosin	Hypovase	500 μg twice daily
Doxazosin	Cardura XL	4–8 mg/day
Alfuzosin	Xatral XL	10 mg/day
Terazosin	Hytrin	2–10 mg/day
Tamsulosin	Flomaxtra MR	400 μg/day

5-alpha-reductase inhibitors

5-alpha-reductase inhibitors are used in BPH to block the conversion of testosterone to another substance, DHT, which appears to stimulate overgrowth of prostate tissue. Side effects include loss of libido, reduced erections and rarely minor breast enlargement.

5-alpha-reductase inhibitor	Brand name	Recommended dose
Finasteride	Proscar	5 mg/day
Dutasteride	Avodart	0.5 mg/day

LHRH analogues

LHRH analogues are used in prostate cancer to 'switch off' testosterone production. They also result in loss of sex drive and in hot flushes.

LHRH analogue	Brand name	Recommended doses
Goserelin	Zoladex	3.6 mg/month or 10.8 mg every 3 months
Buserelin	Suprefact	500 µg three times daily for 7 days
Leuprorelin	Prostap SR	3.75 mg/month or 11.25 mg every 3 months
Triptorelin	Decapeptyl SR	3 mg every 4 weeks

Anti-androgens

Anti-androgens are used in prostate cancer to block the action of testosterone. Side effects include breast tenderness and enlargement.

Anti-androgen	Brand names	Recommended dose
Cyproterone acetate	Cyprostat	100 mg three times daily
Flutamide	Chimax	250 mg three times daily
	Drogenil	250 mg three times daily
Bicalutamide	Casodex	50–150 mg/day

Anticholinergics and antispasmodics

Anticholinergics and antispasmodics are used in BPH to treat irritative symptoms including urinary frequency and urgency. They may cause a dry mouth and blurred vision.

Anticholinergic/ antispasmodic	Brand names	Recommended dose
Flaxovate	Urispas	200 µg three times daily
Oxybutynin	Cystrin	3 mg twice daily
	Ditropan XL	2.5 mg twice daily
Propiverine	Detrunorm	15 mg twice daily
Tolterodine	Detrusitol XL	4 mg twice daily
Trospium	Regurin	20 mg twice daily
Solifenacin	Vesicare	0.5 mg daily

Vasopressin analogues

Vasopressin analogues are used in BPH to reduce the amount of urine produced at night, thus reducing the need to get out of bed to pass urine. They should not be taken with large amounts of fluid and are not advised for men older than 70 years of age.

Vasopressin analogue	Brand names	Recommended dose
Desmopressin	DDVAP nasal	10–20 µg at bedtime
	Desmospray	10–20 µg at bedtime
	Desmotabs	200 µg at bedtime

Other drugs

Anti-inflammatory agents may be given to control pain and inflammation; for example, diclofenac (brand name Voltarol

SR) at a dose of 75–100 mg/day. A wide range of antibiotics may be given to treat infection, such as ciprofloxacin (brand name Ciproxin) at a dose of 500 mg twice daily.

Further information and support

When seeking further information and support, it is important to choose your source carefully. The internet, in particular, is a popular source of material, but sites are unregulated and much of the information is unvalidated and sometimes frankly promotional. The sources listed below are just some of the myriad of books, websites and charities out there, but they should provide further sources of help and information about all aspects of prostate disorders, their treatments and their effects. Although the sources have been put into different groups (and some are listed more than once), there is considerable overlap and the headings are just suggestions as to the best place to look for information first.

General health and lifestyle

- The NHS provides guidance on portion sizes for fruit and vegetables at www.5aday.nhs.uk, or telephone 08701 555455 and ask for a leaflet with details of typical portion sizes.
- Men's Health Forum (www.menshealthforum.org.uk) adopts a number of strategies to improve the health of men and men's health services. One of these is a website called MALEHEALTH (www.malehealth.co.uk), which provides essential, accurate and easy-to-use information about the key health problems that affect men. It also includes an online health check.
- Health of Men (www.healthofmen.com) is a 5-year Big Lottery Fund initiative that provides "quick clear health information for boys and men of all ages". This includes advice about all aspects of lifestyle, such as eating, exercise and dealing with stress, as well as other men's health issues.
- NHS Direct gives a wide range of information about health, conditions, treatments and local services. It can be accessed either by telephone (helpline 0845 4647), via the internet

(www.nhsdirect.nhs.uk) or, if you have digital satellite television, via the NHS Direct Interactive service.

- *The Must-Have Health Guide* is a book by Dr Margaret Stearn that provides down to earth advice on a range of health problems that are difficult to discuss with anyone. Order from www.healthpress.co.uk or telephone 01752 202301, or visit the website at www.embarrassingproblems.com.

- SAGA Health (www.saga.co.uk/health_news) provides broadly based health information for the over-50s. It also includes sections on medicines and supplements, as well as complementary medicine.

Prostate disorders

- Prostate Research Campaign UK (www.prostate-research.org.uk) provides a number of clear, concise and up-to-date leaflets which, in addition to information on every type of prostate disease, include *Sex and the Prostate* and *A Woman's Guide to the Prostate* (all leaflets are free on request). The charity publishes a free quarterly newsletter and has also commissioned a team to précis the latest medical research into layman's terms. Write to: 10 Northfields Prospect, Putney Bridge Road, London SW18 1PE. Telephone: 020 8877 5840. Email: info@prostate-research.org.uk.

- UK Prostate Link (www.prostate-link.org.uk) provides a searchable database of quality-assessed links to prostate cancer information on the internet. Some of the information is quite detailed; for example, there is a link to data on cancer survival in England by Strategic Health Authority. It also has links to a number of sites featuring personal experiences.

- Cancerbackup (www.cancerbackup.org.uk) provides comprehensive information about all aspects of prostate cancer from diagnosis to the latest clinical trials. Write to: Cancerbackup, 3 Bath Place, Rivington Street, London EC2A 3JR. Helpline (staffed by specialist cancer nurses): 0808 800 1234.

- The British Prostatitis Support Association (www.bps-assoc.org.uk) is a web-based organization that offers information and support to sufferers of prostatitis, male chronic pelvic pain syndrome and interstitial cystitis.
- Health Press publishes a number of books by Professor Roger Kirby and others covering prostate disorders. *Patient Pictures: Prostatic Diseases and their Treatments* provides a simple guide to the most common procedures used to treat prostate problems. *Fast Facts: Prostate Cancer* and *Fast Facts: Benign Prostatic Hyperplasia*, although written for doctors, are also read by patients wanting more detailed information. Order from www.healthpress.co.uk or telephone 01752 202301.
- The Prostate Cancer Charity (www.prostate-cancer.org.uk) provides information about all aspects of prostate cancer including diagnosis, treatment and side effects. Write to: 3 Angel Walk, London W6 9HX. Helpline: 0845 300 8383. Email: info@prostate-cancer.org.uk.

Treatment

- Besttreatments (www.besttreatments.co.uk) is run by the *British Medical Journal* with the aim of helping you make better health decisions. It looks at all the best research evidence and decides how well treatments work.
- AstraZeneca Urology (www.prostateline.com) provide a comprehensive site on prostate cancer and its treatment. It also contains a number of links to other relevant organizations worldwide.
- The American Cancer Society (www.cancer.org) provides an online decision tool to help you understand the treatment options for prostate cancer and the possible side effects.
- Bandolier (www.jr2.ox.ac.uk/bandolier) is an independent journal about evidence-based healthcare, written by Oxford scientists. They find information about evidence of effectiveness (or lack of it), and put the results forward as simple bullet points of those things that worked and those that did not.

- The National Cancer Institute in the USA
(www.cancer.gov/prostate), as you might expect, provides
comprehensive information about prostate cancer, but also
includes information and current news about clinical trials
and trial-related data.

Emotional support

- Macmillan Cancerline (www.macmillan.org.uk) has a
good section that puts into words all those feelings that
can be difficult to express. Write to: Macmillan Cancerline,
Macmillan Cancer Relief, 89 Albert Embankment,
London SE1 7UQ. Cancerline: 0808 808 2020.
Email: cancerline@macmillan.org.uk.
- Cancerbackup (www.cancerbackup.org.uk) offers a wide
range of information for both cancer patients, and their
family and friends, covering feelings, relationships and
communication. The website also provides links to local
support organizations by area; go to 'Information', select
cancer type and you will find a list of services including
local support groups. Write to: Cancerbackup, 3 Bath Place,
Rivington Street, London EC2A 3JR. Helpline (staffed
by specialist cancer nurses): 0808 800 1234.

Continence

- The Continence Foundation (www.continence-
foundation.org.uk) offers information, advice and expertise
about bladder and bowel problems, no matter how small. Their
helpline is staffed by a specialist nurse, who will be able to give
you the information and advice you need, and also tell you
where to find your local NHS specialist continence service.
Write to (preferably enclosing a large sae): The Helpline Nurse,
The Continence Foundation, 307 Hatton Square, 16 Baldwins
Gardens, London ECIN 7RJ. Helpline: 0845 345 0165.

Sexuality

- The Sexual Dysfunction Association (www.sda.uk.net) aims
to "help sufferers of impotence (erectile dysfunction) and

their partners". The Association also maintains an index of consultants and others who are competent at impotence management; this information can be accessed by your GP. Write to (send an sae): The Sexual Dysfunction Association, Windmill Place Business Centre, 2–4 Windmill Lane, Middlesex UB2 4NJ. Helpline: 0870 774 3571.

- Sorted in 10 (www.sortedin10.co.uk) offers information about erectile dysfunction and gives advice on approaching your doctor and treatments available, as well as advice for partners on dealing with impotence.

Practical support

- Cancer Support UK (www.cancersupportuk.nhs.uk) helps those affected by cancer to remain in their own home. The website provides details of the help and support available in your area and covers a wide range of issues ranging from financial and housing matters to holidays. The information is also published in several languages.
- Your local library may also be able to provide you with details of services available from your local council.

Support groups

- Macmillan Cancer Support (www.macmillan.org.uk) is just introducing 'Share' columns, where all those affected by cancer can share their experiences.
- Local support groups will enable you to meet others in a similar situation. Your GP surgery may be able to put you in touch with relevant groups. Alternatively, Cancerbackup will be able to put you in touch. Visit: www.cancerbackup.org.uk. Write to: Cancerbackup, 3 Bath Place, Rivington Street, London EC2A 3JR. Helpline (staffed by specialist cancer nurses): 0808 800 1234.
- PSA Rising (www.psa-rising.com) provides information and support for prostate cancer survivors. The site offers online forums and the latest news about prostate cancer and its treatment.

Some medical terms explained

Adjuvant therapy: a treatment that enhances the effectiveness of another therapy.

Advanced: cancer is described as advanced when it has spread beyond the site where it started. Prostate cancer is described as being *locally advanced* when it has invaded parts of the body around the prostate. When the cancer has begun to spread to more distant sites, such as the bones, it is no longer localized and so is referred to as *advanced*.

Alpha-blockers: one of the two types of drug usually prescribed for BPH. They work by helping to relax muscles in the bladder and prostate, which in turn helps to reduce the obstruction to the urinary tract caused by an enlarged prostate.

5-alpha-reductase inhibitors: one of the two types of drug usually prescribed for BPH. They work by blocking the conversion of testosterone to another substance, DHT (see page 117), which appears to stimulate overgrowth of prostate tissue.

Angiogenesis: the development of a blood supply. As a tumour grows, the formation of a blood supply is vital to cancer cells so that they can survive and divide. Researchers are currently developing drugs that could hinder angiogenesis, and so stop cancers growing.

Anti-androgens: drugs that may be prescribed to combat prostate cancer. They work by blocking the action of testosterone, which appears to stimulate the growth of prostate cancer.

Anticholinergic agents: drugs sometimes used to control urinary urgency and frequency associated with BPH.

Benign: non-cancerous. An area of unregulated tissue growth that does not have the capacity to invade surrounding healthy tissue or metastasize is benign.

Biopsy: a sample of tissue taken from the body. Biopsies of prostate tissue are checked in the laboratory for signs of cancer.

Bone scan: a means of seeing whether the cancer has spread to the bones. It involves injecting the patient with a radioactive material that then spreads around the body. The final pattern of distribution will highlight any areas where cancer may be developing.

Botox: Botulinum toxin or Botox is an injectable medicine used extensively by cosmetic surgeons to reduce wrinkles on the face. Recently, early studies have shown that Botox injected into the prostate can improve the symptoms of BPH.

BPH (benign prostatic hyperplasia): a non-cancerous condition that causes the prostate to become enlarged, which may lead to difficulty with urination.

Brachytherapy: a type of radiotherapy for prostate cancer in which radioactive pellets are implanted into the prostate.

Cancerous: refers to unregulated tissue growth that has developed the ability to invade surrounding healthy tissue.

Catheter: a narrow tube inserted into the penis and up into the bladder to drain urine away. A catheter may be inserted during an operation so that the bladder does not fill with urine while the surgeon is working on it. It may be left in place for some time afterwards so that the patient can pass urine while his urethra and bladder heal. Sometimes catheters are also inserted via the penis so that fluid can be passed into the bladder; for example, see urodynamics.

Cavernous nerves: the nerves involved in sexual arousal and erection that lie close to the prostate. They may be disturbed during radical prostatectomy.

Cells: tiny, specialized units from which the body is built. Healthy cells grow and divide as part of their normal lifecycle; in cancer, these processes get out of control because the usual mechanisms that keep them in check have broken down.

Chemotherapy: the use of drugs to destroy cancer cells.

Conformal radiotherapy: a type of radiotherapy that conforms to the shape of the prostate and thereby reduces the radiation dose to nearby tissues.

Continence: the ability to maintain control over bladder and bowel emptying.

CT scanning: a method of using sequential X-rays to build up a three-dimensional picture of the body. CT stands for 'computed tomography'.

Cystoscopy: the use of a telescope to examine the inside of the bladder.

Da Vinci: the name of the robot which facilitates robotic radical prostatectomy.

DHT: the male hormone testosterone can be converted in the body to DHT, which is thought to stimulate the growth of prostate tissue. DHT stands for 'dihydrotestosterone'.

Differentiated (as in 'well, moderately well or poorly differentiated'): a term used to describe healthy, organized tissue. As cancer invades, the tissue structure becomes disorganized or de-differentiated, and looks less and less like normal tissue.

Digital rectal examination: a procedure that allows the doctor to assess the size and texture of the patient's prostate gland. It involves placing a finger into the patient's back passage (rectum) and feeling (palpating) the gland. It is sometimes referred to as DRE.

Gland: a group of cells with the specialized function of making a particular fluid or secretion. The fluid made in the prostate mixes with the jelly-like storage form of the sperm to make semen, which can then be ejaculated.

Gleason score: a number from 2 to 10 that is used as an indicator of how aggressive the patient's cancer is. The score is derived from an assessment (Gleason grade) of two areas of a sample (biopsy) of prostate tissue (e.g. 3 + 4 = 7).

Grade: how the prostate tissue appears under a microscope. The more aggressive the cancer, the less it looks like normal prostate tissue. The Gleason grading system uses a scale of 1–5, with 5 indicating the most aggressive-looking cancer.

Green–light laser prostatectomy: a technique that vaporizes the obstructing prostate tissue to improve urinary flow with minimal risk of bleeding.

HIFU (high–intensity focused ultrasound): a new technique that focuses ultrasound waves on prostate cancer cells. More research is needed before it can be regarded as a mainstream treatment but it does look promising.

Holmium laser enucleation of the prostate (HoLEP): a technique that cuts away the prostate bloodlessly. The tissue is then cut into tiny pieces and removed from the bladder by suction.

Hormones: usually described as 'chemical messengers', these substances can influence processes at different sites in the body. Testosterone is a well-known hormone that influences many aspects of 'maleness'.

Hormone relapsed prostate cancer: prostate cancer that has responded initially to hormone therapy but is beginning to grow again with a consequent rise in PSA values.

Hormone therapy: the use of drugs to block the stimulatory effects of testosterone on the growth of prostate tissue. Technically, orchidectomy can also be described as hormone therapy, as the testicles are removed so that testosterone is no longer produced.

Impotence (or erectile dysfunction): a state in which a rigid erection cannot be achieved and/or maintained.

Intensity modulated radiotherapy (IMRT): a type of radiotherapy that can target high doses of radiation to a very specific area of the body thereby reducing the dose of radiation to normal tissues nearby.

Laser prostatectomy: a new technique to treat obstruction due to BPH that involves almost no blood loss.

LHRH analogues: drugs used in hormone therapy for prostate cancer. They work by switching off testosterone production. LHRH stands for 'luteinizing hormone releasing hormone'.

LUTS: lower urinary tract symptoms. The term used to describe the range of symptoms associated with BPH.

Lymph nodes: these occur at intervals throughout the lymphatic system and act as filters, so cells such as cancer cells tend to accumulate at these points. A well-known example of the lymph nodes (or 'glands') lie in the neck just below the jaw; these tend to become swollen during flu-type illnesses.

Lymphatic system: a network of vessels that drain fluid (lymph) from the body's organs so that it can be filtered and returned to the blood.

Malignant: see Cancerous.

Maximal androgen blockade: the use of LHRH analogues and long-term anti-androgens to help slow the progression of prostate cancer.

Metastases: secondary cancers that occur at sites distant from the original cancer. A cancer has the ability to metastasize when cells can break off from the primary tumour and establish secondary tumours at other sites.

MRI: a means of building up a three-dimensional picture of the body using magnetic fields. MRI stands for 'magnetic resonance imaging'.

Oncologist: a doctor who specializes in the medical treatment of cancer.

Open prostatectomy: an operation for BPH that involves removing the central part of the prostate. Access is gained via an incision through the abdominal wall.

Orchidectomy: an operation for prostate cancer in which both testicles are removed from the scrotum so that testosterone production ceases.

Palliative care: this becomes important in the later stages of cancer where the aim of the medical team is to make the patient pain-free and as comfortable as possible.

Pathologist: a doctor who examines tissue samples microscopically to obtain information to help with diagnosis and treatment.

PCA3: prostate cancer antigen 3. A new and experimental gene-based marker for prostate cancer found in the urine after vigorous massage of the prostate gland.

Pelvic pain syndrome: see prostatodynia.

Perineum: the area around and between the scrotum and anus.

Peripheral zone: the part of the prostate gland in which prostate cancer usually starts to develop. It is also the part that usually becomes inflamed in prostatitis.

Phytotherapy: the use of plant extracts to combat illness, such as BPH.

PIN (prostatic intraepithelial neoplasia): the earliest stage in uncontrolled cell growth. It is not cancer, but is often a forerunner to it.

Prostatodynia: a state in which pain apparently comes from the prostate or surrounding area but there does not appear to be any inflammation or infection.

PSA (prostate-specific antigen): a substance made in the prostate gland that helps to liquefy the jelly-like storage form of sperm. If the prostate tissue becomes damaged or disrupted, as is particularly the case with prostate cancer, PSA leaks out into the bloodstream. As a consequence, blood levels of PSA tend to be higher among men with prostate cancer. A normal PSA value is usually taken as being below 4 ng/mL ('nanograms per millilitre'), but cancer can be present when values are lower than this.

Radical prostatectomy: an operation for prostate cancer in which the prostate, seminal vesicles and a sample of some nearby lymph nodes are removed. It is an option in fit men and only when the urologist believes that the cancer is still confined to the prostate.

Radiotherapy: the use of radiation to kill cancer cells. With external-beam radiotherapy, the radiation is generated from an external source and focused onto the area of the prostate. See also brachytherapy.

Recurrence: when the cancer begins to grow again after a period of dormancy.

Retrograde ejaculation: this occurs following some types of surgery on the prostate. Instead of semen passing out through the penis during orgasm, it passes into the bladder, from which it passes out of the body when the man urinates.

Risk factor: a personal characteristic that increases the likelihood of getting a certain disease. The effect of a modifiable risk factor, such as a high-fat diet or smoking, can be reduced or overcome, in contrast to a non-modifiable risk factor such as belonging to an older age group or having a first-degree relative with the disease.

Robotic radical prostatectomy: a new way of performing a laparoscopic radical prostatectomy that employs the da Vinci robot to achieve 10 times magnification and three-dimensional vision plus very precise dissection of the prostate.

Scrotum: the sac containing the testicles.

Seminal vesicles: storage vessels for sperm. They lie just behind the prostate and may be affected by prostate cancer as it spreads.

Staging system: a method used to assess and describe how far the cancer has spread. The tumour–nodes–metastases (TNM) system is commonly used in the UK.

Testicles (or testes): glands that make sperm and testosterone.

Testosterone: the androgen hormone responsible for the development of many male characteristics. It has a role in stimulating growth of prostate tissue, so some of the drugs for prostate cancer and BPH work by disrupting its production or effect.

Tissue: a collection of cells organized into a structure that performs a specific function.

Transition zone: the part of the prostate in which BPH usually develops.

TRUS (transrectal ultrasonography): an ultrasound method that allows the prostate to be seen. It involves inserting a lubricated ultrasound probe into the rectum, and is often used during brachytherapy and biopsy procedures so that the radiotherapist or doctor can see the exact position of the patient's prostate.

TUIP (transurethral incision of the prostate): an operation for BPH in which small nicks are made in the neck of the bladder and in the prostate to relieve the pressure on the urethra.

TURP (transurethral resection of the prostate): an operation for BPH in which the middle of the enlarged prostate is cut away piecemeal using an instrument inserted up through the penis.

Ultrasound: a method of forming images using high-frequency sound waves.

Ureter: one of two tubes that carry urine from the kidney to the bladder.

Urethra: the tube that runs from the bladder to the tip of the penis, through which urine passes out from the body.

Urodynamics: a test to check how the bladder is functioning and whether the urine flow is blocked. It involves passing a fluid that will show up on X-rays into the bladder (via a catheter) and then recording the movement of this fluid while the patient urinates.

Uroflowmetry (urine flow test): a test to measure the speed of urine output over time. It involves the patient passing urine into a specialized receptacle called a flow meter.

Urologist: a doctor who has specialized in disorders affecting the kidney, bladder and, in men, the prostate.

Vas deferens: a tube that carries sperm from the testis to the prostate gland.

Vasopressin analogues: drugs that may be prescribed to reduce the need to pass urine at night.

Prostate Research Campaign UK needs your help

Much has been achieved in the fight against all prostate diseases since the charity was registered in 1994, but there is still so much more to be done. We need to:

φ fund research into greater understanding and development of new techniques and treatments for all prostate diseases

φ inform and educate men, their partners and their families about prostate diseases

φ inform and train medical professionals, both specialist and non-specialist, in the latest advances in the treatment of prostate diseases

φ create greater awareness about all prostate diseases

φ offer advice, help and hope to those affected by prostate problems.

How you can help

Prostate Research Campaign UK cannot do its work without support. We rely on voluntary donations and fundraising for 100% of our income. There are many ways you can get involved and help us to stop prostate diseases ruining lives.

φ Help to raise money in your local community through a coffee morning, sponsored walk or some other type of fundraising activity or event.

φ Take part in one of our organized events or volunteer to help – more information is available on our website.

φ Set up a regular gift or make a one-off donation online.

φ Leave a legacy in your will to Prostate Research Campaign UK (registered charity number: 1037063).

φ Give shares as a gift and make substantial tax savings on both capital gains and income tax.

www.prostate-research.org.uk

φ Sign a Gift Aid declaration form – using Gift Aid means that for every pound you give, we will receive an extra 28 pence from the Inland Revenue, helping your donation go further without it costing you a single penny. Higher rate taxpayers and companies can also claim tax relief benefits on donations.

Sign up to receive your free copy of our regular newsletter *Update* which has the latest information on research and treatments for all prostate diseases.

Please contact us for any further information on how you can help support the charity.

Prostate Research Campaign UK
10 Northfields Prospect
Putney Bridge Road
London SW18 1PE
Tel: 020 8877 5840
Email: info@prostate-research.org.uk
www.prostate-research.org

Just giving

We have now set up a Prostate Research Campaign UK online fundraising page on the Just giving website. This is an excellent way to donate money securely online. It is extremely easy to use and tax efficient. Visit www.justgiving.com/prostate-research/ to register and set up a sponsorship page complete with your photograph and personal message. Then tell your friends that they can support you via your personal web page, that they can do so securely and with gift aid taken care of (28% tax on every pound donated by UK taxpayers). It can also save you the hassle of collecting sponsorship money.

Index

127

129

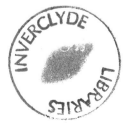